Your Complete Guide to AFib

The Essential Manual for Every Patient With Atrial Fibrillation

Dr. Percy Francisco Morales M.D.

Cardiologist

Electrophysiologist

About the Author

Dr. Percy F. Morales, MD is a board certified cardiologist, electrophysiologist, blogger, and author.

Over the years, Dr. Morales has treated thousands of patients with atrial fibrillation, commonly known as AFib. He likes to say that he knows atrial fibrillation from both the "inside and outside." He has seen firsthand, on a molecular level, the devastating effects of atrial fibrillation from the inside of a patient's heart. While performing catheter ablation procedures on patients, he has seen in detail the intense scarring from AFib as well as the difficulty in reversing the damage done by this serious disease. In addition, Dr. Morales knows atrial fibrillation from the outside as well. He has treated many AFib patients for years at a time, and he sees firsthand how atrial fibrillation affects the daily lives of many patients.

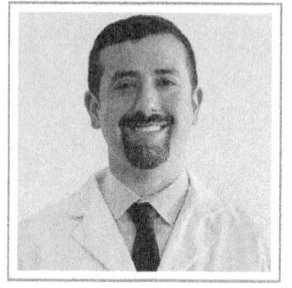

In 2018, Dr. Morales extended his expertise on AFib by creating his blog entitled Dr. AFib. Through his blog he creates evidence-based educational content in an easy to understand format to help patients answer their questions about atrial fibrillation. Through his blog, Dr. Morales has now helped over 150,000 patients across the globe with their atrial fibrillation. Dr. Morales believes that an educated patient results in an empowered patient that will seek better options and treatments.

For many people, there is a path for improved symptoms, reduced risk of stroke, and disease reversal from atrial fibrillation. Hopefully this book can help you find your path for better treatment.

For more information you can visit his blog at: https://drafib.com

Disclaimer

Copyright © Year 2020

All Rights Reserved.

No part of this eBook can be transmitted or reproduced in any form including print, electronic, photocopying, scanning, mechanical or recording without prior written permission from the author.

While the author has taken utmost efforts to ensure the accuracy of the written content, all readers are advised to follow information mentioned herein at their own risk. The author cannot be held responsible for any personal or commercial damage caused by misinterpretation of information. All readers are encouraged to seek professional advice when needed.

This e-book has been written for information purposes only. Every effort has been made to make this eBook as complete and accurate as possible. However, there may be mistakes in typography or content. Also, this eBook provides information only up to the publishing date. Therefore, this eBook should be used as a guide - not as the ultimate source.

The purpose of this eBook is to educate. The author and the publisher do not warrant that the information contained in this eBook is fully complete and shall not be responsible for any errors or omissions. The author and publisher shall have neither liability nor responsibility to any person or entity with respect to any loss or damage caused or alleged to be caused directly or indirectly by this eBook.

See My Full Disclaimer Here: https://drafib.com/full-disclaimer

See My Full Terms And Conditions Here: https://drafib.com/terms-conditions

Dedication

This book is dedicated to my wife Madeline.

Thank you so much for never-ending support.

Preface

In 2018, I started on a path to educate patients about the most prevalent and growing heart arrhythmia across the world, atrial fibrillation. When I first started my blog over two years ago, I was shocked to see little to no patient educational information written by a doctor with experience in managing this serious heart condition. As you can imagine, Dr. Google has never had the responsibility of taking care of a patient face-to-face.

Although there are many articles online written about AFib, many are written by industry professionals. The writers of these articles usually do not have the experience of sitting face-to-face with a patient with atrial fibrillation and managing their health for years at a time.

I frequently tell people that starting my blog gave me a new way to listen. As I developed a following, I noted how countless people were not receiving proper communication when it came to treatment options for AFib. Atrial fibrillation can be a very confusing condition with many different treatment options. I strive to provide patients with a better understanding of their treatment options, as well as educate patients on how lifestyle modifications can also significantly improve AFib.

Now, with my complete guide, I wanted to bring patients with AFib an all-encompassing assistant to help them become empowered patients when it comes to AFib. I truly believe that an empowered patient will receive the best care and get the best outcomes. No matter if you are newly diagnosed with atrial fibrillation, or if you have had AFib for years, you will find something of benefit for you here.

If you have been recently diagnosed with atrial fibrillation, it may be overwhelming to figure out what this all means for you. You may struggle to find the right answers to your questions online, and I hope this guide will help you start your treatment on the correct path.

If you have struggled with atrial fibrillation for years, this book can be of service to you as well. I will outline several treatment options, but also give my personal insight on what works best in individual circumstances. Hopefully this book will help you find the missing pieces of the puzzle to get better AFib treatment.

How To Use This Guide:

This guide is broken down into multiple sections. Take a look at what is most pertinent to you first, but I would strongly encourage you to read the whole guide to get a bigger picture of atrial fibrillation and treatment options. Over time, understanding multiple treatment options may make a significant difference in your care.

The guide starts off with a thorough discussion about atrial fibrillation. Here I will explain the science behind atrial fibrillation, what causes it, and explain the progression of AFib. Understanding the progression of AFib is a key point to understanding treatment options and the success rate of various treatment options.

Next, I will discuss what I feel is the most important first step for AFib treatment, stroke risk reduction. Here I will discuss why atrial fibrillation increases risk of stroke and show you how to calculate your individual risk for stroke. I will also discuss treatment options which can include medications and procedures.

In the next section, I will discuss foods and other items which can trigger atrial fibrillation. Understanding your individual triggers can make a major impact in reducing symptoms. Here I will also emphasize the lifestyle modifications that can improve and sometimes even reverse atrial fibrillation.

Your Complete Guide to AFib

Following that, I will discuss a wide variety of treatment options for atrial fibrillation. AFib can be improved through a variety of options which can include medications, lifestyle modifications, as well as procedures.

Lastly, I'll discuss future treatment options for AFib and help you set up an AFib Action Plan for your own care.

Are You Ready To Get Started?

Table of Contents

Introduction 11
What Is Atrial Fibrillation? 12
The Prevalence of Atrial Fibrillation 14
What Causes Atrial Fibrillation? 16
The Natural Progression of Atrial Fibrillation 17
    How To Slow Down the Progression of Nonvalvular AFib 20
    How To Slow Down the Progression of Valvular AFib 21
Paroxysmal Atrial Fibrillation 21
Persistent Atrial Fibrillation 24
Chronic Atrial Fibrillation 25
Atrial Fibrillation and Risk for Stroke 27
    How Does AFib Increase Risk for Stroke? 27
    How To Determine Your Individual Risk of Stroke With the CHADSVASc Risk Score Calculator 29
    The Link Between AFib and Cryptogenic Stroke 31
    Reducing Risk of Stroke With Blood Thinning Medications 33
    Reducing Risk of Stroke With Procedures 36
Determine Your Trigger For AFib 39
    How Diet Can Be a Trigger For Atrial Fibrillation 39
    Caffeine 40
    High Sodium 40
    High Sugar Foods 41
    Trans Fat 42
    Gluten 42
    Magnesium and AFib 43
    Potassium and AFib 46

The Link Between AFib and Alcohol 48

Smoking and Atrial Fibrillation 50

Exercise and Atrial Fibrillation 56

Sleep Apnea and AFib 61

Does Stress Affect AFib Symptoms? 64

The Truth Behind Weight Loss and Reversal of Atrial Fibrillation 65

What Are Common Treatment Options for Atrial Fibrillation? 67

    Common Medical Therapy for AFib 67

    Blood Thinning Medications for Stroke Risk Reduction 68

    Heart Rate Controlling Medications 68

    Heart Rhythm Controlling Medications 70

Cardioversion for AFib 72

Ablation Procedures for AFib 76

    Traditional Catheter Ablation for AFib 77

    Surgical Ablation Procedures 83

    The Mini Maze Procedure 83

    The Hybrid or Convergent Procedure 86

    The AV Node Ablation 87

How Are Pacemakers Used for the Treatment of AFib? 88

Natural Treatments for Atrial Fibrillation 91

Special Circumstances 93

    Patients With Both Atrial Fibrillation and Coronary Artery Disease 93

    Patients With Both Atrial Fibrillation and Congestive Heart Failure 96

    The Athlete With Atrial Fibrillation 97

    Young Patients Diagnosed With Atrial Fibrillation 99

The Future of AFib Treatment 100

    Home Monitoring Devices for Atrial Fibrillation 100

Implantable Cardiac Devices 100
KardiaMobile 103
The Apple Watch 106
Future Directions for Treatment Options 108
Create Your AFib Action Plan 112
Conclusion 118

Introduction

Atrial fibrillation or AFib is a condition of the heart that can increase the risk of heart failure, blood clots, strokes and other related complications. AFib itself refers to an irregular heartbeat that patients suffer from due to this common arrhythmia. The heart is not able to pump blood efficiently since the upper chambers of the heart quiver rather than contract effectively together.

With AFib, patients can have very different experiences. Some feel no symptoms and find out about this condition after a checkup. Meanwhile, others experience painful symptoms like a rapid heartbeat, shortness of breath, weakness, light-headedness, skipped beats, or feelings of an irregular heart rhythm.

No matter what symptoms you experience, it is essential to educate yourself about this condition to bring it under control. If left unchecked, it can lead to worsening symptoms, increase the risk for several complications such as stroke, and decrease quality of life.

As a cardiologist and electrophysiologist, I have had the honor of helping thousands of patients suffering from this growing heart condition. Having treated thousands of patients over the years, I am in a unique position to help you with this condition, its symptoms, complications, and what can be done to improve AFib.

By reading this eBook, you will have the core knowledge that every AFib patient needs. You will understand the treatment options that are available as well as their success rates. You will also know what happens as the disease progresses and what steps you can take to mitigate the negative consequences and to slow progression. This eBook provides all of the basic knowledge that you need to know about this condition, the fundamental knowledge that I wish every patient with AFib knew.

This guide is meant to educate you about AFib in simple language that is easy enough for anyone to understand. I explain key topics about AFib in the simplest possible terms so that you can learn quickly about this condition and empower yourself as a patient.

AFib does not mean that you should live with symptoms for the rest of your life. You can educate yourself about steps you can take to control and potentially improve this condition. In some cases, AFib can even be reversed if the proper steps are taken. This eBook serves as a guide that can help you towards this end.

Please note that this guide is simply meant to inform and is in no way an alternative for professional medical treatment. Your doctor can give you the best advice and treatment options depending on your individual condition. There are many factors to consider, including a patient's past medical history, when deciding on an optimal treatment plan. Do not attempt any kind of self-diagnosis or treatment on your own. Always keep your doctor informed and discuss with your doctor before making any changes mentioned in this guide.

With this in mind, you are now ready to go through this comprehensive guide about AFib. Let's make a positive impact on your AFib and overall health together.

What Is Atrial Fibrillation?

Atrial fibrillation refers to a medical condition in which the heart beats irregularly. It is a type of arrhythmia. Think of an arrhythmia as an electrical disease of the heart. Due to a short circuit or misfire, your heart is not working the way it should be during a natural heartbeat. Instead of pumping blood with sufficient force, all in unison, the upper chambers of your heart are simply quivering. Your blood cannot circulate properly when this happens. AFib increases the risk of several complications including heart

Your Complete Guide to AFib

failure and stroke. In any arrhythmia, the heart may beat too fast, too slowly or irregularly. AFib is the most common type of arrhythmia affecting millions across the world. More and more patients are diagnosed with new atrial fibrillation every day.

With atrial fibrillation, the upper chambers of your heart are unable to provide the pumping strength needed to get your blood throughout your body. Instead of circulating properly, blood may start pooling in the upper chambers of your heart, also known as the atria. The risk of clot formation will increase due to this pooling and it leads to an increased risk of stroke.

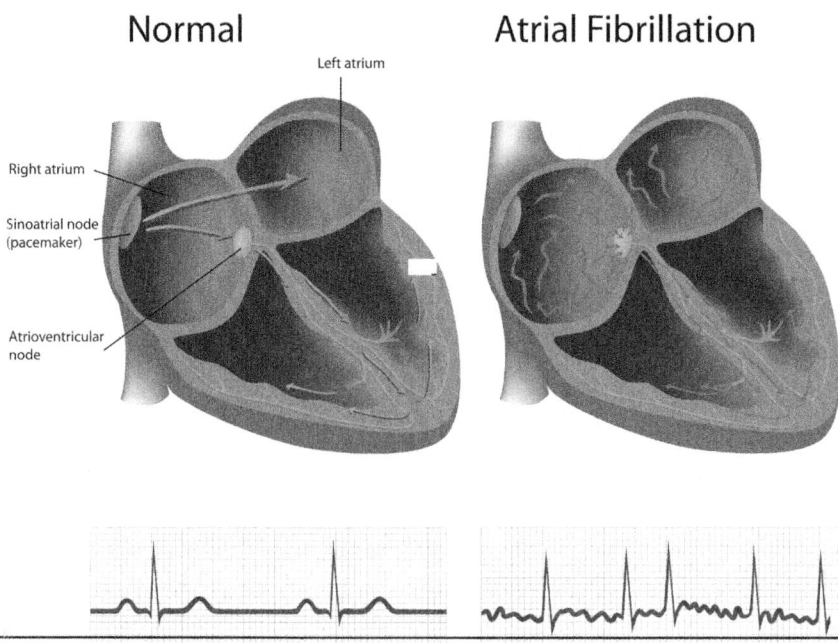

During AFib, the steady normal heartbeat is replaced by the rapid, chaotic beats of atrial fibrillation.

Here is how the heart normally functions. First, the top chambers of your heart squeeze blood; these are the atria. Then, the lower chambers of the heart pump blood; these are the ventricles. The timing of these contractions is absolutely crucial for effective pumping of blood. If there is a mismatch in timing, then the heart cannot pump blood effectively the way it should. This is exactly what happens during AFib. With AFib, the electric pulses that drive contractions of the atria and ventricles get out of sync. Instead of working together correctly, the upper chambers are not squeezing blood at all. During AFib, the upper chambers of the heart can be quivering very fast, at a rate of over 600 beats per minute. Fortunately, the pulse comes from the lower chambers, or ventricles. Although the ventricles will not usually go as fast as the atria does during AFib, it is not uncommon to see heart rates from 100 to 200 beats per minute.

AFib can occur in brief episodes that stop on their own called paroxysmal atrial fibrillation, and it can also happen continuously, which is called persistent atrial fibrillation. I will further discuss stages of atrial fibrillation in more detail later in this book.

For More Information:

1. Fantastic animation further demonstrating the rapid activity of a heart during atrial fibrillation: *https://www.youtube.com/watch?v=y_DeCe5r_To*

The Prevalence of Atrial Fibrillation

According to the CDC, the number of people in the US with atrial fibrillation ranges from 2.7 million to 6.1 million. It is expected that as the population ages, the prevalence of atrial fibrillation will continue to increase.

The CDC also states that the incidence of AFib for people under 65 years of age is 2 percent. However, for people over 65, the incidence of AFib then rises to 9 percent. There is a very strong age-related association with the diagnosis of AFib.

During 2017, atrial fibrillation was mentioned as one of the causes of death in over 166,000 death certificates. In over 26,000 death certificates during the same period, AFib was stated as the main cause of death.

AFib occurs more commonly in people of European descent as compared to African Americans. However, African Americans with AFib have a greater risk for developing complications associated with the condition, like heart failure, heart disease and stroke.

Atrial fibrillation is one of the few types of heart disease that is actually increasing in prevalence. More and more people are diagnosed with AFib every day. But why is this happening? A quick explanation is that people are living longer than ever before. There are more people in their 70s and 80s, and still living active lives, than ever before. In addition, people are living longer with heart disease due to advances in treatment for heart disease. It is not uncommon to see someone with a past heart attack still alive and doing well some 20 years after their heart attack. As you will see, advanced age and past history of heart disease are some of the strongest risk factors to eventually develop AFib.

For More Information:

1. CDC website on atrial fibrillation: https://www.cdc.gov/heartdisease/atrial_fibrillation.htm

What Causes Atrial Fibrillation?

Damage to the heart and long-term medical conditions are the most common causes of atrial fibrillation. The likelihood of suffering from AFib increases with the following medical conditions:

- High Blood Pressure
- Diabetes or Metabolic Syndrome
- Obesity
- Heart Failure - also known as CHF
- Congenital Heart Defects
- Coronary Artery Disease
- Hyperthyroidism
- Family History of AFib
- Sleep Apnea
- Chronic Kidney Disease
- Chronic Lung Disease

Despite the multiple causes of atrial fibrillation listed above, there are some groups of patients that are at risk for higher complications from this disease. AFib is linked to higher mortality rates in people who have past cardiovascular conditions or who have undergone heart surgery in the past. AFib also leads to greater mortality in people with a history of stroke and heart failure.

Certain lifestyle choices may also be associated with a higher incidence of AFib. Alcohol consumption is a significant risk factor, particularly abuse of alcohol. Tobacco use has also been associated with an increased risk for AFib. In addition, mental health conditions and elevated stress levels are also linked to a greater risk of having AFib.

Age is another important risk factor for AFib. The incidence of AFib increases significantly with age. People between the ages of 65 and 85 represent the majority of AFib cases. The main reason for the significantly increased risk with age is thought to be due to age related fibrosis. Not unlike the way someone gets wrinkles as they age, the heart can develop an increasing amount of scar tissue in the upper chambers of the heart as people age. This increasing scar tissue is what causes age-related fibrosis which then significantly increases risk for AFib.

Lastly, men have a higher incidence of AFib. But as women in general tend to live longer than men, the total number of women and men with AFib is about the same, statistically speaking.

The Natural Progression of Atrial Fibrillation

Atrial fibrillation can start and stop sporadically. However, it may then progress to a stage where it will become more sustained or persistent and ultimately permanent. For most people, AFib will progress to more persistent stages if nothing is done. Fortunately, there are multiple treatment options to reduce this progression, and in some cases reverse AFib, as you will see in this book.

There are rare times where AFib may just stop by itself. There may be times where AFib was caused by a single medication or isolated event and stopping the medication or recovering from an event will prevent AFib recurrence. However, in most cases, it is a long-term medical condition, especially if nothing is done to treat or reverse the condition. In addition, even though there may be examples of isolated causes of AFib, most people who develop AFib also have the most common risk factors for AFib listed above.

AFib is usually categorized into two different types: valvular versus nonvalvular AFib. Valvular AFib is due to defects of a heart valve, most commonly the mitral valve. Nonvalvular AFib is the result of long-term health conditions such as smoking, diabetes, high blood pressure and other factors besides the valves. Most of the time, for nonvalvular AFib, patients have had common risk factors such as high blood pressure or diabetes for several years before AFib develops. Both kinds of AFib are progressive in nature. That is, as time goes on, the condition will become worse if nothing is done. Episodes of AFib will likely happen more frequently and last longer as time progresses. But don't be discouraged, there are multiple ways to slow or reverse this progression as I will discuss in this book.

When AFib is first diagnosed, it will usually come and go and episodes will stop on their own. However, as the years go by, the condition will deteriorate, episodes will last longer and pose greater problems if nothing is done. How quickly the condition deteriorates is known as the rate of progression. The rate at which AFib advances can have a strong impact on your health.

However, understanding the rate at which AFib is progressing is challenging because it is difficult to quantify its progression and symptoms for some people. Doctors still don't have an accurate way of predicting progression for an individual patient.

In the vast majority of cases, AFib will get worse if nothing is done. The reason for this is that the disease will do more and more damage to your heart as time goes by. This is due to a common phrase that many AFib experts say: "AFib begets AFib." What this means is that AFib causes structural damage to your heart tissue and likewise causes problems with the heart's electrical and mechanical functions, which then leads to more AFib. The damage caused by AFib on your heart muscle will continue to get worse over time if nothing is done.

Most people, when first diagnosed with AFib, have paroxysmal atrial fibrillation. Paroxysmal AFib is defined as atrial fibrillation where the episodes of AFib do not last longer than one week. This is typically seen in people newly diagnosed with this condition. However, the condition may become more persistent rather quickly. After about a year, many people find that their AFib episodes have become more persistent, or more frequent, and may last in excess of one week.

Some people experience a rapid deterioration in their condition. For others, the decline may be more gradual and may take several years.

To prevent AFib from getting worse too fast, you should get early treatment and follow your doctor's instructions diligently. Besides just heart rate control, treatment should also focus on rhythm control since restoring the heart rhythm back to normal often results in slower progression of this condition. Lifestyle modification also plays an essential role in limiting progression of AFib and in its reversal.

To slow down the progression of AFib, you must take control of risk factors linked with this condition. For example, high blood pressure, congestive heart failure, and atherosclerosis can make the condition worse much faster. Uncontrolled diabetes is another key risk factor that can accelerate the worsening of AFib. Hyperthyroidism can also quicken progress of the condition. And drinking alcohol can certainly make your AFib much worse faster.

There are also other health issues where a faster rate of progress is often observed. People with a faster resting heart rate and those with an enlarged left atrium of the heart experience a quicker rate of AFib progression.

If you have suffered a stroke, have sleep apnea, or are obese, then AFib will likely progress at a faster rate if left untreated.

Researchers are continuing to investigate the role of inflammation, kidney disease and fibrosis (gradual scarring and thickening of tissue) in the progression of AFib.

How To Slow Down the Progression of Nonvalvular AFib

Most people living with AFib have nonvalvular AFib. Fortunately, there are more ways of managing and treating it when compared to valvular AFib.

Most patients when diagnosed will have paroxysmal atrial fibrillation, where episodes come and go and stop on their own. In this earlier stage, medications may not be needed right away. But you can and should make lifestyle changes and make better health choices if you wish to slow down the progression of nonvalvular AFib.

To slow down progression of AFib, your doctor might recommend you quit smoking, consume a heart-friendly diet, eliminate alcohol, exercise more, and lose weight if you are overweight. You will have to avoid food ingredients that can trigger AFib episodes. These can include alcohol, caffeine, and processed foods. You may also have to avoid cold medicines, especially ones that contain stimulants. Hesitating to act upon these lifestyle recommendations may make your AFib worse more quickly.

Persistent AFib can be more difficult to treat since it is a more advanced form of the condition. Patients frequently need medications or other kinds of treatment like an ablation or cardioversion to treat or potentially reverse this type of AFib. I will further discuss these treatment options later in this book. The combination of treatments that will work best for you depends on many factors, like your overall health, the length of time you have had AFib, and your age.

When a cardioversion or medications fail to bring results, you may have to consider a catheter ablation. This method of treatment works with intense heat or cold energy to create strategic scars in the parts of the heart which are causing AFib. I will further discuss procedures for AFib in detail later in this book.

How To Slow Down the Progression of Valvular AFib

Catheter ablation and rhythm control medication can be helpful for the treatment of valvular AFib as well, especially in earlier stages. Lifestyle modifications can also be extremely beneficial for patients with less severe valvular disease. These can be useful options for patients with mild to moderate valvular disease. However, for patients with more severe valvular disease, such as severe mitral regurgitation, surgical repair or replacement of the valve will provide much greater relief from atrial fibrillation than lifestyle modification, medical therapy, or even a catheter ablation.

If your health permits and you need open heart surgery for other medical conditions (for instance, repairing a faulty heart valve), your doctor might recommend the maze procedure. Similar to a catheter ablation, this procedure, done as an open heart surgery, makes use of intense heat energy to generate scars that may help to bring misfiring under control. Performing a maze or a mini-maze surgery is a common treatment option for AFib patients with valvular heart disease who need surgical repair of a heart valve.

Paroxysmal Atrial Fibrillation

In paroxysmal atrial fibrillation, people experience symptoms of AFib that may come and go and stop spontaneously. The episodes are sporadic in nature and can start and stop on their own without any regular pattern.

Here are the most common symptoms of paroxysmal atrial fibrillation:

• Heart Palpitations: feelings of a noticeably rapid, strong, or irregular heartbeat

• Fatigue

• Lightheadedness or Dizziness

• Shortness of Breath

• Overall Weakness

It is possible to experience the aforementioned symptoms over the course of a few days, for a few seconds, and anywhere in between the two extremes. The symptoms typically do not last for more than seven straight days to be defined as paroxysmal atrial fibrillation.

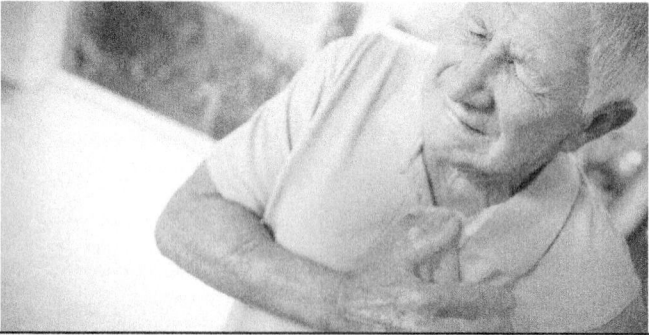

Paroxysmal atrial fibrillation can result in sudden debilitating symptoms.

People with paroxysmal AFib tend to experience an erratic heartbeat and other symptoms for a relatively short time period (not exceeding seven days), after which their heart rhythm reverts to normal. For people who have symptoms that last for over seven days, this is referred to as persistent atrial fibrillation, which I will further discuss below.

Although paroxysmal atrial fibrillation is typically less severe than other stages of AFib, there are many patients who suffer severe, debilitating symptoms from sudden episodes of AFib. In addition, paroxysmal AFib can quickly progress to the next stage, persistent atrial fibrillation, if not treated and managed properly. The AFib symptoms may then become more severe, frequent and/or persistent as the condition deteriorates.

If you have paroxysmal atrial fibrillation, it is imperative to seek treatment early to ensure that it does not progress into more serious stages. About 10 to 30 percent of patients with paroxysmal atrial fibrillation progress towards persistent atrial fibrillation after about a year. The rate of progression depends on many factors such as obesity, hypertension and age.

Around 40 percent of all patients with AFib suffer from paroxysmal AFib.

In general, younger people have a higher likelihood of presenting with paroxysmal atrial fibrillation at the time of diagnosis. Meanwhile, older people have a higher risk of developing the more advanced form of AFib, persistent atrial fibrillation, at the time of diagnosis.

You might be surprised to know that even endurance and "elite" athletes are at higher risk of paroxysmal atrial fibrillation. One explanation for this could be the enormous strain that grueling long-distance runs have on the heart. There have also been studies that have demonstrated that endurance athletes can develop more scarring or fibrosis in their atrium, which may explain the increased risk for atrial fibrillation in this population.

Persistent Atrial Fibrillation

Persistent atrial fibrillation is the progression of AFib from paroxysmal atrial fibrillation to a more serious and persistent form. Persistent AFib is still treatable, but it is much more difficult to treat or reverse when compared to paroxysmal atrial fibrillation. On the other hand, persistent AFib is less difficult to treat and manage than the permanent or chronic forms of atrial fibrillation, depending on the duration of persistent atrial fibrillation. In general, the longer someone is in persistent AFib, the harder it is to reverse it. It much harder to reverse persistent atrial fibrillation that has been present for 10 months than one that has been present for three months.

In persistent atrial fibrillation, a person may begin to experience the similar symptoms of paroxysmal atrial fibrillation more frequently and for a longer duration than paroxysmal atrial fibrillation. Symptoms may include heart palpitations, shortness of breath, or fatigue. For many patients, these symptoms can be more subtle than those with paroxysmal AFib, but the symptoms will typically continue to build up and become more noticeable. There are frequently times when someone gets diagnosed with new persistent atrial fibrillation, and they have likely been in consistent AFib for several weeks.

Although there are many patients that get diagnosed with new atrial fibrillation when they are in persistent AFib, in most cases the AFib is not new for the patient. On questioning patients, they will usually give a history of palpitations or flutters for years, but AFib was not officially diagnosed until it became persistent.

You should also keep in mind that persistent atrial fibrillation can also be asymptomatic. That is, you might never experience any symptoms at all; there are many patients with persistent AFib that get diagnosed accidentally during a regular checkup.

Your Complete Guide to AFib

In my opinion, asymptomatic persistent atrial fibrillation is one of the most dangerous types of AFib. When someone does not notice any symptoms, it is hard for them to appreciate the long-term risks that are still faced with AFib. Some of these patients are reluctant or noncompliant with medications including blood-thinning medications, which will then lead to a significantly increased risk for stroke.

Chronic Atrial Fibrillation

Chronic atrial fibrillation is now commonly referred to as a long-standing persistent AFib under the new guidelines. As the name suggests, long-standing, persistent atrial fibrillation is AFib that is ongoing for a long time period. If AFib lasts for more than 12 months, then the AFib is typically classified as long-standing persistent AFib. This kind of AFib is continuous and does not easily respond to medication or procedures for disease reversal.

The symptoms that you may experience owing to long-standing, persistent AFib are the same as those for paroxysmal and persistent AFib. One major problem with chronic AFib is that it becomes very difficult to reverse and restore the heart's natural rhythm.

To diagnose a patient with chronic AFib, it would usually require several office visits and several cardiac tests such as an external cardiac monitor that can be worn for several weeks. In addition, there are structural changes in the heart that can be seen on an echocardiogram (ultrasound test of the heart) which can also help a doctor diagnose a patient with chronic AFib.

Doctors frequently treat chronic AFib aggressively to mitigate the risk of a blood clot. For patients with chronic atrial fibrillation, the treatment goals are frequently rate control to make sure your average heart rate is acceptable, and blood thinning medications to reduce risk of stroke. Treatment options to restore normal rhythm, including catheter ablation, usually have a very low success rate in patients with chronic or long-standing persistent atrial fibrillation.

Medications for rate control are typically the first line of treatment for chronic atrial fibrillation in order to improve the average heart rate. Commonly used rate controlling medications include digitalis, calcium channel blockers and beta blockers. I will discuss options for medical therapy with more detail later in this book.

For most patients, your doctor will prescribe blood-thinning drugs for reducing the risk of developing blood clots. Examples of these drugs include rivaroxaban (XARELTO), dabigatran (Pradaxa), edoxaban (Savaysa), apixaban (ELIQUIS), heparin and warfarin (Coumadin). I will discuss blood thinning medication in more detail later in this book.

If your condition cannot be brought under control through medications alone, then you might have to undergo invasive medical procedures. One of these is a cardioversion, which works by reverting your heart rhythm to normal rhythm with a low voltage electric current. Another method is a catheter ablation in which a strategic scar is made to reduce AFib and to restore your heart rhythm to normal. Again, for patients with long-standing persistent atrial fibrillation, most procedures with the intention to reverse atrial fibrillation, such as a cardioversion or traditional catheter ablation, will have a low success rate.

For patients with chronic AFib, another type of ablation performed is called an AV node ablation. This type of ablation is performed to control the heart rate in combination with a pacemaker. The goal of the AV node ablation is not to cure AFib but to control it, patients are still in AFib after this type of ablation. After an AV node ablation, patients are dependent on a pacemaker for all their heartbeats. The heartbeat is nice and steady but comes at a cost of being dependent on a pacemaker device for every heartbeat, forever. This type of procedure may sound extreme, but it can be an excellent option for some patients with chronic AFib who clearly cannot tolerate or are not doing well on medical therapy.

In general, atrial fibrillation progresses from paroxysmal to persistent and then long-standing or chronic atrial fibrillation if nothing is done. As atrial fibrillation continues to worsen, the success rate of rhythm control strategies to restore normal rhythm becomes lower and lower. However, with early treatment, you can see a significant reversal of AFib.

Atrial Fibrillation and Risk for Stroke

How Does AFib Increase Risk for Stroke?

Atrial fibrillation is a disorder of the heart that impacts its rhythm. The upper chambers of the heart, the atria, are quivering instead of beating normally. Due to this quivering of atrial fibrillation, the heart has difficulty pumping blood effectively. As a result, the blood will start to pool in the upper chambers of the heart where it might turn into blood clots.

In the upper left chamber of the heart, called the left atrium, a blood clot may develop. If it breaks loose, it might reach the brain where it can impede blood flow, which then leads to a stroke. In a similar way, blood clots from the heart can hinder the flow of blood to other organs as well. However, since there is a significant percentage of blood that goes to the brain with every heartbeat, any blood clot in the heart has the highest chance of going to the brain and leading to a stroke.

Not everyone with AFib has the same risk for stroke. Age is an important risk factor that plays a central role in the likelihood of a stroke from AFib. The older a patient is, the higher is the risk for stroke. There is a major increase in risk for stroke when a patient is over 75 years of age. Other conditions that can increase the odds of suffering from a stroke as a result of AFib are diabetes, high blood pressure, coronary artery disease, and congestive heart failure.

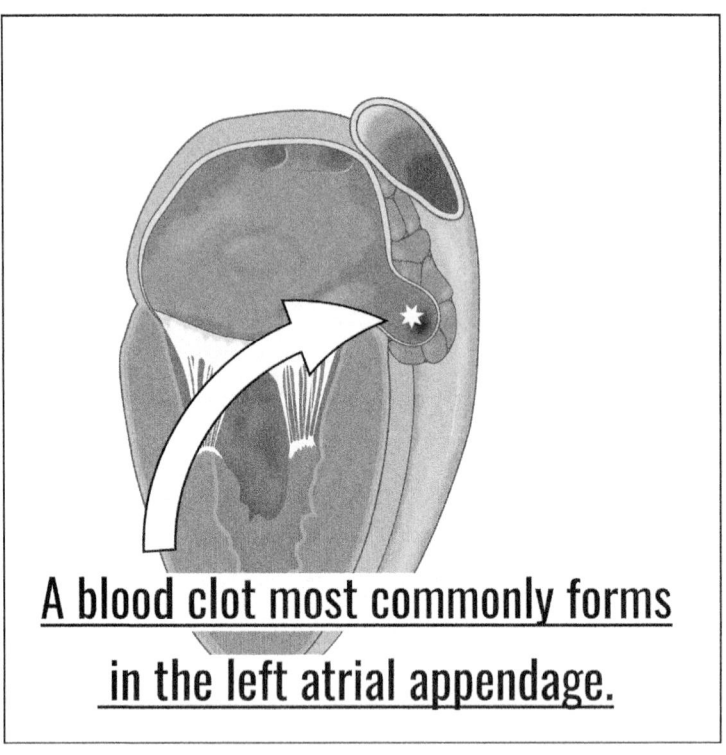
A blood clot most commonly forms in the left atrial appendage.

Another major risk factor for stroke in patients with AFib is a past history of stroke. Statistically speaking, once someone has had a stroke, the risk for having a second stroke is significantly increased.

To reduce the risk of blood clots, doctors often prescribe blood-thinning drugs that are known as anticoagulants. Commonly prescribed blood thinners include warfarin, Rivaroxaban (brand name XARELTO), Edoxaban, Dabigatran and Apixaban (brand name ELIQUIS).

In case you cannot tolerate standard recommended blood-thinning medications, your doctor may recommend a procedure known as left atrial appendage closure, especially if you are considered a patient at increased risk for a stroke. This procedure involves sealing the left atrial appendage which is a small sac located in the left atrium. I will further discuss a left atrial appendage closure procedure in more detail later in this section.

You can also adopt several lifestyle choices to cut down the risk of having a stroke due to AFib. This involves heart-friendly choices like avoiding alcohol, quitting smoking, maintaining healthy weight, consuming foods that are good for the heart and regular exercise. It is imperative to keep cholesterol levels and blood pressure under control. Controlling high blood pressure and diabetes are both very important to reduce your risk for stroke from AFib.

How To Determine Your Individual Risk of Stroke With the CHADSVASc Risk Score Calculator

Since AFib substantially increases your risk of stroke, your cardiologist may want to assess your individual risk for stroke. As I mentioned before, not everyone with AFib has the same statistical risk for stroke. Your doctor will typically assess your individual risk for stroke using the commonly used CHADSVASc risk scoring system.

The CHADSVASc risk score is a risk assessment method that takes into account several risk factors that influence your chance of getting a stroke due to AFib. The CHADSVASc score ranges from 0 to 10 with a higher score indicating a higher risk of stroke from AFib.

The CHADSVASc score is calculated based on the following risk factors:

- Congestive Heart Failure
- Age

- High Blood Pressure
- Gender
- Peripheral Vascular Disease
- Previous Stroke or Blood Clot
- Diabetes

Points are awarded to calculate the score based on the above risk factors. The weightage varies according to the importance of the factor. Since age, previous stroke and blood clot status are very important, two points are awarded for ages above 75 years and also for a previous incident of stroke. If your age is between 65 years and 74 years, then only one point is awarded. Congestive heart failure, high blood pressure, diabetes, peripheral vascular disease and being female all carry one point each.

With a higher CHADSVASC score, there is a statistically greater chance for suffering a stroke. This score is essential as it can help your cardiologist determine your individual chances of having a stroke. Based on this probability, your doctor may prescribe the right course of treatment and suggest recommendations to lower your risk.

There are certain steps you can take to reduce your risk of stroke if you have AFib. Suppose you have a family history of diabetes and you are still free from this medical condition. You can take steps to minimize your chances of getting diabetes in the future. For instance, you can adopt a healthy diet and incorporate a daily exercise routine according to your doctor's instructions to lower your risk of developing diabetes.

If you have high blood pressure, is crucial to control it and thus lower your risk of stroke from AFib. Based on your condition, your doctor may prescribe blood pressure medication and lifestyle changes to bring down your blood pressure. Although frequently medications are needed to improve high blood pressure, there are many lifestyle modifications that also significantly improve blood pressure. Losing weight and reducing daily salt intake can significantly improve high blood pressure and reduce risk for stroke.

Fortunately, a person's CHADSVASc score is not permanent. You can actually lower your CHADSVASc score, and thus risk of stroke, by adopting a healthy lifestyle. Using lifestyle modifications, you may be able to reduce your stroke risk by losing weight and eliminating high blood pressure, or diabetes for example. Although not directly measured in the CHADSVASc score, quitting smoking can also significantly reduce your risk for stroke.

The Link Between AFib and Cryptogenic Stroke

Cryptogenic stroke (CS) is a cerebral ischemia (or stroke) whose origin is not known. In simple terms, it means that doctors are unaware of the cause of the stroke. CS causes may not be easy to determine since they require exhaustive testing. About a third of all ischemic strokes can be classified as cryptogenic.

Pinpointing the exact factors behind CS is not simple. Even after extensive testing, including MRIs and testing for blockages in arteries of the neck, there may still be no clear information from which to draw a conclusion. Even a heart test like an echocardiogram or wearing a heart monitor may be unable to uncover a cause. Some stroke patients who come to hospitals for treatment may not find out the cause of their stroke before they are discharged from the hospital.

The reason for many cases of CS is undiagnosed AFib. There is an important reason why pinpointing the CS causes is difficult. Since detecting AFib can be very tricky, especially when episodes come and go, locating the root cause of CS may be difficult if undiagnosed AFib is the main cause.

AFib is one of the leading causes of CS. However, to be sure that AFib is indeed the cause, the doctor has to detect an AFib episode to be completely certain. Due to the sporadic and unpredictable nature of paroxysmal AFib, as I discussed previously, diagnosing AFib can be quite difficult at times. A CS patient suspected of having paroxysmal AFib may spend several days in the hospital without having any AFib episode that their doctor can detect. Hence, the risk factor behind CS may remain inconclusive and obscure.

According to research conducted in this area, it may take up to 80 days of continuous heart monitoring for doctors to detect AFib as the CS cause, if it is indeed a factor. Hence, doctors often recommend further testing for their CS patients after they are discharged. CS patients need to undergo testing and monitoring once they leave the hospital to uncover AFib to see if it is the cause behind the stroke. Being fully certain about AFib being the cause of the CS episode is crucial for proper diagnosis and the right course of treatment. After a proper diagnosis of AFIb, a patient can be started on proper treatment, such as blood-thinning medications, to reduce the risk of future stroke.

After leaving the hospital, patients that have just recovered from a CS event may need to wear an external heart monitor. The heart monitor is a device that can check for undiagnosed AFib. However, these heart monitors may be worn for usually no more than a month. As such, they may not be able to pick up AFib. As explained, 80-days monitoring may be necessary to detect AFib in some studies.

Another solution can be an implantable cardiac monitor. These heart monitoring devices go under the skin and can stay operational for up to three years. These devices are about the size of a paperclip and are quickly inserted under the skin in the chest, right over the heart. These devices usually only take a few minutes to place. They can provide a much better chance of diagnosing AFib as a possible factor. If you have suffered from a cryptogenic stroke, check with your doctor if an implantable cardiac monitor is the right treatment for you. Commonly used implantable cardiac monitors at the time of this writing include the Medtronic Linq and the Abbott Confirm Rx.

Reducing Risk of Stroke With Blood Thinning Medications

Atrial fibrillation patients have a substantially higher risk of stroke compared to the general population. Thankfully, blood thinning medications, also known as anticoagulants, can substantially bring down the risk of stroke.

As discussed previously, the heart is not able to pump blood effectively due to atrial fibrillation. Blood starts pooling in the upper heart chambers, where a blood clot may form. This clot may travel towards the brain where it can hinder blood flow and cause a stroke. Since blood thinners reduce the risk of blood clot formation, they are a useful treatment option for stroke prevention. Doctors often prescribe anticoagulants to their AFib patients so that the risk of blood clot formation and consequent stroke is significantly reduced.

However, some patients who have atrial fibrillation may not take these medications since they have no effect on how they feel. Patients do not notice any significant change to their wellbeing as a result of taking anticoagulants. Blood thinners for AFib do not stop or reduce AFib episodes, they are purely for stroke risk reduction. This fact, coupled with other factors like the risk of bleeding and the costs involved, is why many people with AFib may give up taking anticoagulants.

In general, the benefits of blood thinning medications for AFib patients outweigh the risks involved. Anticoagulants may, in fact, cause bleeding and other side effects in some cases. This overall disadvantage is much less significant in comparison to the risk of death, disability, permanent brain damage and paralysis due to stroke for some patients.

In recent years, the FDA has approved newer blood thinners that may be safer and more effective than warfarin, a traditional blood thinner used for several decades. Four blood thinners have been approved in the past few years. These include: edoxaban (Savaysa), apixaban (ELIQUIS), rivaroxaban (XARELTO) and dabigatran (Pradaxa). While these drugs have been approved in the last few years, the classic anticoagulant drug warfarin has been used for around 60 years as a blood thinner. Warfarin was studied in several clinical trials during the 1990s and was found to significantly reduce risk of stroke from AFib when compared to Aspirin.

These newer blood thinning medications have certain key differences between them. The main problem with warfarin is that it can react with certain foods and medications so that the risk of bleeding becomes greater or the effectiveness of the drug goes down. Hence, periodic blood tests are necessary to ensure that patients are within the recommended therapeutic range of warfarin. The newer medications, on the other hand, are known to have fewer interactions. They also do not need frequent blood monitoring. For most patients, the standard dose provides steady, therapeutic blood thinning effects. For some patients, such as those with abnormal kidney function, a lower dosage of these medications is recommended.

Anticoagulants reduce the risk of ischemic strokes, that is, strokes instigated by blood clots formed in the heart. Unfortunately, due to their blood thinning effects, they may increase the risk of stroke due to bleeding in the brain. This type of stroke is known as a hemorrhagic stroke. Fortunately, the newer blood thinning medications carry a smaller risk of hemorrhagic stroke when compared to warfarin. The newer blood thinning medications have a lower risk for both kinds of strokes, those due to blood clots (ischemic) and those due to bleeding (hemorrhagic).

Another key advantage of the newer blood thinning medications is the speed at which they work. Warfarin can be quite slow in this regard. It takes a few days for warfarin to manifest its blood-thinning effects. In addition, it can also take a few days for the effects of the medication to subside after patients stop taking warfarin.

The newer drugs, on the other hand, are much quicker. Their effects can start almost immediately, usually within a few hours, when patients start taking them. Their effects can also subside rapidly when patients stop taking these drugs. Usually these newer blood thinners completely wear off within about two days. This is a key advantage that can prove to be a lifesaver.

For any surgery or procedure, it is necessary for the effects of blood thinning medication to subside. The blood thinning effects of warfarin do not subside quickly unless a reversal agent is given. But with the advent of newer anticoagulants, the blood thinning effects can subside rapidly so patients can undergo surgery whenever it is needed.

Patients who experience life-threatening bleeding from anticoagulants, or those that need emergency surgery, may need reversal agents that can immediately nullify the blood thinning effects of anticoagulants. For warfarin, the preferred blood thinning reversal agent is vitamin K.

Other reversal agents are now approved for the newer blood thinners as well. For instance, Praxbind is now approved as a reversal agent for Pradaxa. Praxbind may be needed for emergencies in the rare situation where the life-threatening bleeding from Pradaxa cannot be controlled, or emergency surgery is needed. At the time of this writing, reversal agents for newer blood thinners such as ELIQUIS and XARELTO have been recently approved as well. These new reversal agents are all intravenous and fairly expensive, they are usually only used during very severe or life-threatening bleeding, or if needed prior to emergency surgery. In addition, at the time of this writing, the availability of reversal agents for ELIQUIS and XARELTO may be limited.

Reducing Risk of Stroke With Procedures

The WATCHMAN is a procedure that can serve as an alternative for stroke risk reduction for patients with atrial fibrillation (that is not due to a heart valve issue) who are unable to tolerate standard blood thinning medications. There are many patients who are unable to tolerate standard recommended blood-thinning medications for a variety of reasons. Reasons may include major bleeding (significant bleeding in your stool or urine for example), increased risk for falls, or history of severe anemia. The WATCHMAN device has emerged as a viable alternative under specific circumstances for people who are unable to tolerate warfarin or other blood-thinning medications. Your doctor can assess your health condition to ascertain whether or not WATCHMAN is feasible for you.

About four out of five AFib patients are willing to try an alternative to anticoagulants for reducing their risk of stroke. About one third of AFib patients worry about the possibility of a stroke and the side-effects posed by blood thinning medication.

The WATCHMAN device is a permanent heart implant that is shown by studies to substantially reduce the risks associated with strokes in nonvalvular AFib patients. The magnitude of stroke risk reduction is comparable to taking a blood thinner like warfarin, but without all the long-term bleeding risks. After undergoing the WATCHMAN procedure, the overwhelming majority of patients can stop taking warfarin after just 45 days. Hence, the WATCHMAN device can give a patient freedom from the lifelong use of warfarin or other blood-thinning medications for AFib. Thus, you may avoid the risk of major bleeding and other side effects associated with the long-term use of these medications.

How It Works:

The WATCHMAN works by reducing the risk of stroke associated with atrial fibrillation. As you already know, the pooling of blood in the LAA (left atrial appendage) leads to clots that can cause strokes.

This is particularly true for nonvalvular AFib patients since over 90 percentof strokes from AFib are due to clots that develop in the LAA. Hence, sealing off this portion of the heart can reduce the risk of stroke for many patients, especially those who are unable to tolerate standard blood-thinning medications.

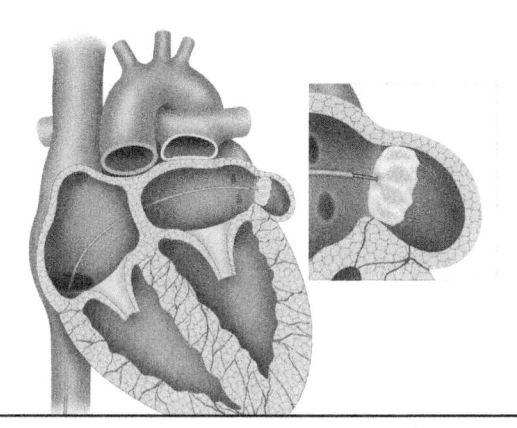

A Watchman Device seals off the left atrial appendage, where blood clots typically form during AFib.

The WATCHMAN implant is designed so that it fits inside the LAA. The implant works by completely sealing off the LAA and preventing blood clots there.

The Procedure:

The WATCHMAN device is installed through a one-time procedure. The implant is permanent, so it does not require any additional procedures.

The WATCHMAN implant is inserted via a needle puncture in the vein in your upper leg. The surgeon inserts a thin tube much like an ordinary stent procedure. The implant is then guided towards the LAA where it is placed. The procedure is typically completed in an hour and usually requires general anesthesia. Patients typically stay overnight in the hospital and are allowed to leave the following day. Once the WATCHMAN procedure is completed, you will still be prescribed a blood thinner like warfarin for 45 days or until the LAA is completely sealed off.

A WATCHMAN device can serve as a feasible alternative for reducing the risk of stroke in AFib patients. The WATCHMAN device is very well studied with several years of clinical trials behind it. More than 90,000 patients across the globe have WATCHMAN implants. Over 10 clinical trials have yielded positive results on the device's effects on the risk of stroke in AFib patients.

Long-term studies have proven that the WATCHMAN device is effective for reducing the risk of stroke in nonvalvular AFib patients. Not only can the device alleviate the risk of strokes, it can also reduce mortality and disabling strokes, and decrease risk for major bleeding episodes.

Overall, I feel that the WATCHMAN procedure is an excellent option for patients with increased risk for stroke due to AFib who are unable to tolerate standard, recommended blood-thinning medications. Many patients continue to struggle with clinically significant major bleeding due to blood thinning medications that can be significantly reduced with a WATCHMAN procedure. In addition, there are many patients with increased risk of stroke that are currently off of blood-thinning medications due to history of bleeding, thus leaving them unprotected from an increased risk of stroke. At the time of this writing, the WATCHMAN is the only approved catheter-based, left atrial appendage closure procedure. However, I know that there are alternative left atrial appendage closure devices under study, so there may be more options available in the near future.

For More Information:

1. Online calculator to determine your individual risk for stroke from atrial fibrillation: *https://clincalc.com/Cardiology/Stroke/CHADSVASC.aspx*

2. Crystal AF Study demonstrating link between cryptogenic stroke and atrial fibrillation: *https://www.nejm.org/doi/full/10.1056/nejmoa1313600*

3. Learn more about the WATCHMAN procedure: *https://www.watchman.com/en-us/home.html*

Determine Your Trigger For AFib

How Diet Can Be a Trigger For Atrial Fibrillation

AFib patients need to be careful about certain foods that are not heart-healthy. There are even some otherwise heart-healthy labeled foods that may not be recommended for AFib patients due to the unique health conditions of atrial fibrillation.

In general, foods that are bad for your heart can subsequently aggravate your AFib. Hence, they should be avoided strictly or at least minimized so that the risk can be alleviated. Typically, this includes high fat foods as well as foods that contain a lot of sugar and sodium. I also frequently advise patients to avoid processed foods with artificial sugars or flavorings as much as possible. Too much of these foods can exacerbate your AFib and even heighten your risk of a heart attack or stroke, as well as contribute to obesity and inflammation.

Caffeine

Does caffeine trigger your AFib? For years, the standard advice has been to avoid caffeine if you have AFib. This means avoiding beverages like coffee, tea, guarana, and soda.

As far as studies go, the results are mixed. Clinical studies do not show a clear link between AFib and caffeine intake. In addition, a recent study showed coffee was possibly beneficial for AFib patients. However, when I counsel my patients, I usually tell them one cup of coffee a day is fine as long as it does not appear to trigger any AFib episodes. In general, I feel that coffee or tea is a healthier drink for caffeine then any soda due to soda's added sugars and artificial flavorings.

Given the mixed results, it might be safer to minimize caffeine, especially if it is a clear trigger for your AFib. You should definitely avoid high-caffeine beverages like energy drinks, which are also typically high in sugar.

High Sodium

It is typically recommended to consume less than 2,300 mg of sodium a day, meanwhile the average American eats 3,400 mg a day. I like to give people a visual for daily salt intake: 2,300 mg of sodium is approximately one teaspoon of salt a day.

Foods with high sodium, such as processed lunch meats, may trigger AFib episodes. Excess salt in your diet will likely also raise blood pressure. Increased blood pressure may then also trigger an AFib episode. So, avoid sodium saturated foods like pizza, canned soups, and fried foods, as much as possible. Make low sodium foods a regular part of your diet by staying away from processed foods which generally contain excess salt.

Keep this in mind, more than 70 percent of the sodium that Americans eat comes from packaged, prepared, and restaurant foods. In general, adding salt to your food is a relatively low quantity of salt compared to the sodium content already found in processed and packaged foods. You are much better off with fresh foods and trying to season them yourself. In addition, you can try non-salt seasonings like garlic or onion.

High Sugar Foods

High sugar foods can lead to obesity, inflammation, and high blood pressure. High blood sugar can then trigger AFib episodes. So, check the label on that bottle of your favorite pasta sauce or ketchup you eat. Look for the added sugar in the foods you have been eating. Artificial sugars can be just as bad or even worse, in my opinion, than traditional sugar. I am a strong believer that natural sugar in low quantities is much better than low calorie, artificial sweeteners.

The American Heart Association recommends a daily intake of no more than 36 grams of sugar (9 teaspoons) for men, or 25 grams (6 teaspoons for women). Recent studies have shown that the average American consumes around 77 grams of sugar a day. To put it in perspective, one can of Coca Cola has 39 grams of sugar, more than the daily recommended amount of sugar.

Choose to eat foods in their most natural state. I frequently tell my patients to keep their food closest to the way it came from the ground or animal. The less processed the food is, the better. When you know where your foods come from, you know no one added any extra flavorings that could trigger AFib.

In 2016, foods labels changed to include added sugars. This is a very important part to look it on any of your processed foods or beverages. The natural sugars in a food may be ok, but it is the added sugars that significantly increase the total carbohydrates in a product. When cooking at home, attempt to replace or reduce sugar, consider alternative sweeteners like cinnamon, nutmeg, vanilla, ginger or lemon.

Trans Fat

It is important to avoid the consumption of trans fat as it is a proven risk factor for a wide array of chronic diseases. Trans fats are the most dangerous kinds of fat and you should do your best to avoid them. Unfortunately, doing so is easier said than done. After all, trans fats are ubiquitous and are among the main ingredients of processed foods as they extend shelf life and are economical.

Many kinds of processed foods, including fried foods, doughnuts, potato chips, cookies, crackers and other packaged items, contain trans fat. If you come across processed foods, then chances are they have trans fat. Make sure that you read labels carefully. If you find partially hydrogenated vegetable fat or margarine listed in the ingredients, then that food has trans fat.

Gluten

Another matter to look out for is gluten intolerance. Gluten is a kind of protein that can be found in grains like barley, rye and wheat. It is commonly found in products like pastas, breads, condiments, and many kinds of packaged foods. Gluten intolerance is rather unfortunate since gluten appears to be everywhere.

If you are allergic to wheat or have gluten intolerance, then your body may react adversely in response to consumption of products having gluten. You may suffer from a higher level of inflammation due to gluten, which is a risk factor for many kinds of chronic diseases. In addition, having gluten intolerance may lead to malabsorption of essential vitamins and minerals, a concept sometimes referred to as a "leaky gut."

It may be no coincidence that gluten-containing foods such as bread and pasta are also foods that contain high sugar and sodium contents. I frequently tell patients that bread and pasta are the most common processed foods that people eat. As a result, reducing gluten-containing foods can significantly improve your health and AFib, even if you don't have a true gluten intolerance.

Magnesium and AFib

There is an abundance of promotional content and anecdotes that laud the effects of magnesium on AFib symptoms. But is it a magic pill as some sources would like you to believe? What does the science say about magnesium supplements for AFib patients? Is there any evidence to show AFib benefits from magnesium supplements in the long term?

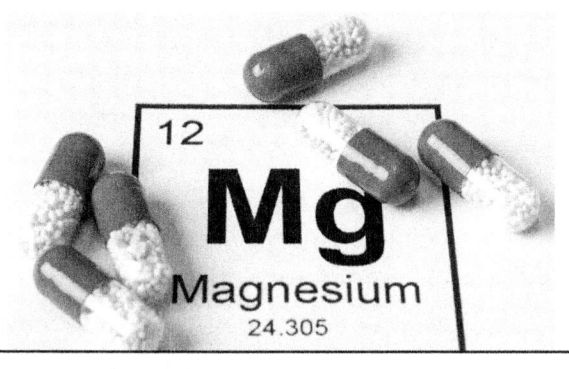

Does Magnesium supplementation help with AFib?

To begin with, most people in the US do not get enough magnesium through their diet. The standard American diet, which is low in whole grains and leafy green vegetables, is also low in magnesium. This is alarming because magnesium has a central role in regulating biochemical processes and enzymes in your body. Magnesium is critical for your heart rhythm and it is a key substance for energy production. Only around 1 percent of your total magnesium is present in your blood at any given time. The rest is present in your non-muscular soft tissue, muscle and bone mass. During a typical test for magnesium deficiency, however, it is the blood levels of magnesium that is measured.

There is some research to suggest an association between AFib and low magnesium levels. In the Framingham Heart Study, those with the lowest magnesium levels had the greatest risk of AFib. The study was done on 3,500 subjects over the course of two decades.

Another study also shows similar results. Analysis of an HMO database in 2016 suggested a higher AFib risk for those with slightly low blood magnesium levels.

Although the data does suggest that low magnesium is probably associated with AFib risk, there is no long-term study to indicate that magnesium supplements are of any help in treating AFib. There are some clinical studies that explored the effects of magnesium on atrial fibrillation, but not only are they small and short term, they were done specifically in the hospital in the settings of heart surgeries.

AFib episodes present a serious risk to patients recovering from open heart surgery. It can lengthen recovery and prolong the hospitalization for such patients. About 10 studies have been published with regards to the effect of magnesium on reducing risk of post-operative AFib for patients who have undergone open heart surgery. The overall results are inconclusive. There is no consensus on how magnesium supplements aid recovery in post-open heart surgery patients with some studies showing slight improvements, while some show no effect.

There are also a number of studies that look at the effect of magnesium infusions on emergency room care and recovery. These studies showed that magnesium infusions can help to slow down a heart rate that is too high because of an AFib episode, as a rate controlling medication. Magnesium also helps improve the success rate of a cardioversion (an electrical shock to the heart) when used in conjunction with other anti-arrhythmic medications.

In theory, magnesium tests could be more accurate if they measured body tissue levels instead of blood levels since the overwhelming majority of magnesium is stored in your tissues. While a number of tests are available that measure body tissue magnesium levels, these tests may not be covered by insurance. To carry out these tests, you may have to pay out of your own pocket. As a result, the blood test for magnesium is what is most commonly used to test for magnesium deficiency.

How to Supplement with Magnesium

There are several magnesium supplement brands that specifically target heart patients claiming that their products can improve heart problems. This advertising is directed towards AFib patients as well.

The first thing to realize is that the absorption rate is different for the various forms of magnesium. Another important point to consider is whether or not these magnesium supplements are of any help to AFib patients.

In addition, the FDA does not regulate magnesium supplements much like other supplements. There is no data from scientific studies to suggest that magnesium supplements can improve AFib symptoms.

If you have AFib, then you should get your blood magnesium levels tested. If you want to save money, then getting blood magnesium levels is the better option since it is usually covered in health insurance plans. The other type of blood magnesium testing is more expensive and you may have to pay out of pocket. A commonly used test for measuring magnesium levels inside of your cells is called the RBC Magnesium test.

If the test shows a deficiency in magnesium, then you should include more magnesium rich foods into your diet. These can include fatty fish, nuts, legumes, bananas, avocados and dark green vegetables. You can then incorporate magnesium supplements into your diet if needed.

One of the cheapest and most widely available options for magnesium supplementation is magnesium oxide. You can find it in most drug stores and the supplement is typically easily tolerated.

But depending on your specific health conditions, you may benefit more from alternative magnesium supplements such as magnesium taurate or magnesium glycinate. In addition, there are some specialty magnesium supplements that contain a combination of magnesium products. Most of these alternative magnesium supplements are not available in a typical drug store. You may find them in specialty vitamin stores or online. To find out about the ideal magnesium supplement for you, always check with your doctor.

There are some patients I have met in person as well as online that swear that magnesium supplements significantly improved their AFib symptoms. While magnesium supplements may help some, there is no doubt that lifestyle changes, dietary choices and weight loss can have a more powerful effect on your AFib condition. There are several studies showing how lifestyle modifications can bring significant improvements and disease reversal in AFib patients. So, instead of simply relying on supplements alone, you should also think of a holistic and comprehensive strategy involving multiple key factors.

Potassium and AFib

Potassium has an important role to play in the regulation of heart rhythm and heart muscle contraction. Low or even high levels of potassium can trigger heart arrhythmias like AFib.

Low potassium levels may be the result of poor dietary intake or some medications. Frequently used diuretic medications, used for either high blood pressure or as a fluid pill for congestive heart failure can lead to low potassium levels. Stronger doses of diuretic medications, such as lasix, frequently require potassium supplementation.

You can eat the following natural foods to increase potassium levels in your body if you are found to be deficient:

- Fruits including oranges, apricots, bananas and avocados
- Prunes
- Tomatoes
- Root vegetables like beets and sweet potatoes
- Squash

Before making your diet potassium-heavy, you should discuss it fully with your doctor since high amounts of potassium might interfere with certain pharmaceutical drugs. Patients with chronic kidney disease should always discuss with their doctor any potential increases in potassium intake.

For More Information:

1. Study demonstrating safety of caffeine in AFib patients: https://www.acc.org/latest-in-cardiology/articles/2018/04/16/16/27/is-caffeine-safe-protective-for-patients-with-afib-arrhythmias

2. Magnesium for AFib, Myth or Magic? https://www.ahajournals.org/doi/full/10.1161/CIRCEP.116.004521

The Link Between AFib and Alcohol

Wine, especially red wine, is touted for its supposed health benefits and popular science would have you believe that a glass or two of red wine a day is good for your heart. However, the science on this is quite complicated. While content platforms on the internet casually publish studies that indicate possible benefits to heart health, they may look the other way whenever a major study arises that gives results to the contrary. You should be skeptical about any alleged benefits of alcohol and red wine with respect to heart health, especially when it comes to AFib. The science on this topic is far from conclusive and there are contradictory results.

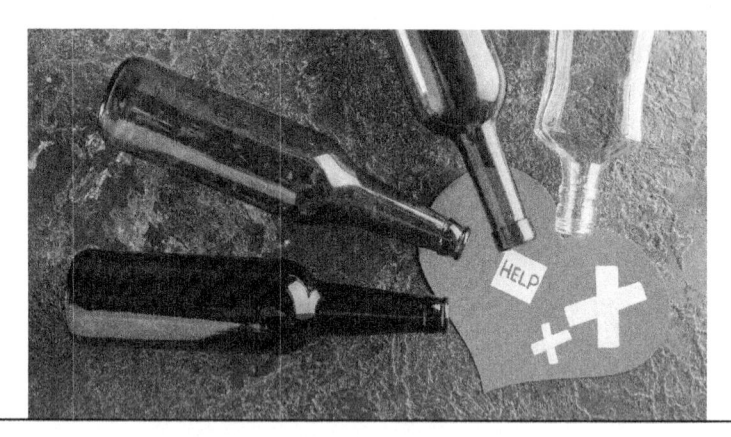

Alcohol and AFib do not mix

While there is a controversy as to the effects that alcohol and red wine have on those with healthy hearts, there appears to be less controversy with respect to AFib.

The link between excessive alcohol intake and AFib can be seen in a phenomenon that is informally known as the "holiday heart syndrome." Emergency rooms across the country usually see an influx of patients with AFib episodes during the holidays due to the deleterious effects of alcohol on heart health. Although many cases of AFib attacks occur during binge drinking, there is evidence to suggest that these attacks may also occur 12 to 36 hours after the binge drinking event.

While it should be fairly obvious that regular binge drinking will no doubt worsen AFib, there appears little doubt now that even lower quantity, moderate alcohol consumption of no more than a drink per day can also worsen symptoms in AFib patients if they do not give up drinking or significantly reduce usage.

One recent study from 2016 shows that even low levels of alcohol consumption can be detrimental to those with atrial fibrillation. The systematic review concluded that people who do not give up alcohol would progress more quickly from paroxysmal to persistent atrial fibrillation. Alcohol users were also observed to suffer from more AFib episodes even after an ablation procedure.

This goes against conventional wisdom, which suggests that small amounts of alcohol may be beneficial for the heart. The results show very convincingly that AFib and alcohol are not compatible.

Another recent study was performed to investigate the effects of frequency since all too often, current guidelines, recommendations and studies pertaining to alcohol are based on the absolute amount of the substance rather than the frequency of use.

Based on the results of the study, reducing the frequency of alcohol use is also important besides controlling the absolute amount.

In this recent study, the analysis indicated that an increase in alcohol consumption raises the risk of developing AFib. In this study, there was a 2 percent increase in the risk of new-onset AFib per each gram of alcohol consumed per week. Hence, even a slight increase in absolute alcohol consumption by just one drink a WEEK can raise AFib risk. This certainly challenges the notion that moderate alcohol consumption is "good" for the heart.

This study also demonstrated that the number of drinking sessions per week is an important risk factor for new-onset AFib that was independent from the total amount of weekly alcohol intake. Patients who drink every day represented the highest risk group and those who drink once per week were the lowest risk group for new-onset AFib in this study. Based on these findings, it shows that even frequent drinking of small alcohol servings is detrimental for your heart rhythm and increases risk of AFib. In addition, it was noted that drinking frequency leads to sleep disturbance which is also a well-established risk factor for AFib.

For more information:

1. Alcohol and atrial fibrillation, a sobering review: https://www.sciencedirect.com/science/article/pii/S0735109716364695

Smoking and Atrial Fibrillation

Nicotine from cigarettes can certainly make AFib worse. Smoking is known to be very damaging for the heart and blood vessels. Smoking is also known to raise the risk of heart disease, heart attack, and stroke. You should consider giving up smoking completely to slow down the progression of heart disease including AFib. Your doctor may recommend nicotine replacement or some other smoking cessation medicine so that you can successfully quit smoking.

Chronic exposure to nicotine is a well-established risk factor for heart failure, myocardial infarction and atherosclerosis. In addition, there are also studies that provide evidence of smoking causing atrial fibrillation. In a 2018 study, it was found that smoking could also be a significant risk factor for developing atrial fibrillation. This meta-analysis study took the combination of several different studies together and analyzed over 600,000 patients. The study found that there is a significant increase in the risk of atrial fibrillation for people who smoke.

People who smoked in this study had a 32 percent increased risk for developing atrial fibrillation. Even former smokers still had a 9 percent increased risk for developing atrial fibrillation.

One of the most significant points noted from this study was not just that smoking by itself causes atrial fibrillation, but the amount that people smoked further increased the risk for developing atrial fibrillation. Overall, the more that someone smoked the higher the risk of developing atrial fibrillation. For example, for someone who smoked 10 cigarettes a day their risk of developing of atrial fibrillation was 17 percent. For 20 cigarettes a day it was 32 percent, and if you smoked 30 cigarettes a day that risk went up to 45 percent for developing atrial fibrillation! There was a significant increase in risk for developing AFib for every 10 cigarettes that you smoke a day.

In addition, there is evidence that patients with AFib who also smoke have a higher risk for stroke, disabling stroke, or recurrent strokes. As you can see, smoking not only increases the risk of getting AFib, but also increases the risk of disabling complications such as stroke.

Is it the cigarettes themselves or the effects that cigarette smoking can also have on someone's body that increases risk for atrial fibrillation? The answer to this is unclear. Smoking can influence atrial fibrillation, but it also increases risk for people developing lung conditions such as COPD and emphysema. Smoking also increases risk for heart disease, such as coronary artery disease and high blood pressure which can also influence risk for developing atrial fibrillation. In addition, there have been studies in the past that showed that nicotine itself can also increase fibrosis, or scarring of the heart, which can also cause atrial fibrillation.

To understand the dangers posed by smoking, you have to put the dangers of cigarettes in context by looking at the statistics. The sobering statistics make it clear that smoking will do no good for your heart health. In addition, smoking is one of the biggest causes of preventable death in the US and many parts of the world.

In the US alone, smoking kills around 480,000 (almost half a million people) every year, according to the Centers for Disease Control and Prevention. Smoking kills more people each year than all firearm incidents, motor vehicle accidents, alcohol abuse, illegal drug use and HIV infection deaths put together. Smoking accounts for 80 percent of deaths from chronic obstructive pulmonary disease.

Also, it is not just the nicotine alone that is responsible for the deleterious effects of cigarette smoking on heart health and AFib symptoms. There are several other toxic compounds in cigarette smoke, including carbon monoxide and tar, that can harm your heart in many ways and worsen AFib symptoms. These harmful chemicals result in the accumulation of plaque within arteries that can obstruct blood flow and also injure the delicate lining inside blood vessels. As a result, cigarette smoking frequently leads to atherosclerosis. These compounds also worsen cholesterol profile and adversely affect fibrinogen levels (a blood-clotting substance). These factors can then increase the risk of stroke for patients with AFib.

Long term cigarette smokers will likely want to know if there are any safe levels for smoking. Unfortunately, smoking is so damaging for health, and heart health in particular, that there is no such thing as "safe smoking." Smoking is a dose-dependent risk factor for several chronic diseases including heart disease and the risk of AFib. That is, the more you smoke, the greater your risk of developing these medical conditions. If you smoke less, then the chances of developing these chronic diseases will be less, but it will never come down to zero unless you quit smoking.

Your Complete Guide to AFib

The only way to bring down the risks posed by smoking is to give up smoking completely. You should not think that light smoking will not damage your heart or not worsen your risk of AFib. You will experience some amount of heart damage with even light smoking.

You can gain several benefits from not smoking. Your AFib symptoms will not progress as quickly as they would if you continue to smoke. You might even experience fewer AFib episodes if you give up smoking as many former smokers have discovered to their pleasant surprise. You can add several years to your life, improve your senses of taste and smell, have more energy for work and exercise, improve the appearance and health of your skin and teeth, and above all, greatly reduce your risk of developing high blood pressure, heart disease, and stroke.

All that being said, quitting smoking is hardly an easy task. However, with the right mindset, determination, and tactics, it can be done. Countless others have done it before you and so can you. The good news is that ex-smokers typically enjoy a much better quality of life without smoking. In fact, many former smokers feel much better off without it as you will soon discover for yourself.

Here are the tactics that you can follow to give up smoking and prevent your AFib from getting worse:

- Set a deadline. You can pick a special day like your birthday or wedding anniversary.

- Get rid of all cigarettes and tobacco products from your workplace, car and house. Also discard all ashtrays, matches and lighters.

- Keep away from your triggers. You must know what compels you to smoke. Does being hungry increase your craving for smoking? Or perhaps high stress levels? You should think of alternatives. For instance, if it is hunger, then you should think about having a healthy fiber-rich snack. If it is stress, then you can practice stress reliever techniques like deep breathing, meditation, stretching, walking and even power napping.

- Tell your coworkers, friends and family that you have made up your mind to quit smoking. For those who smoke, insist that they do not smoke in front of you.

- When you do plan to quit, inform your doctor about it because nicotine or the lack thereof, can affect pharmaceutical drugs that you might be using. Your doctor might want to make some changes to your medications if you quit smoking.

- You should talk to your doctor about medications, nasal sprays, lozenges, tablets, inhalers, patches or gums that can help you to cease smoking. These products can help you to avoid cigarettes when you feel the urge to smoke. They are also very helpful for reducing withdrawal symptoms.

- Go for counseling or a group program that assists people in giving up smoking. Prescription medicines, nicotine alternatives and group therapy are a powerful combination that has helped many to quit smoking. The success rate for medications is better when they are used along with group sessions.

You should know that withdrawal symptoms will be less pronounced with nicotine replacement and medications. Withdrawal symptoms will also go down with the passage of time as you continue to refrain from smoking. Always discuss with your doctor if nicotine replacement is the right treatment for you.

No matter how strong the withdrawal symptoms, you should know that you are doing your health immense good by ceasing smoking.

The longer you go without cigarettes or other tobacco products, the greater the health benefits. Since many of these benefits are related to heart health, you are bringing down risk factors that worsen AFib as well. The US Department of Health outlines the following health benefits that you gain with the passage of time as you continue to abstain from smoking:

- Heart rate goes down within just 20 minutes of giving up smoking.

- After 12 hours of cessation, carbon monoxide levels in the blood return to normal.

- After three months, the risk of heart disease and heart attack goes down substantially and lung function improves.

- After a year, the risk of coronary heart disease due to smoking is slashed by half compared to an active smoker.

- Five years later, your risk of stroke is the same as that of a nonsmoker.

- Ten years later, your lung cancer death risk is half that of a smoker.

- Fifteen years later, your risk of heart disease and coronary artery disease is around the same as someone who does not smoke.

Quitting smoking is always a good decision. By remaining off tobacco, the risk factors for AFib, heart disease and stroke go down considerably and even normalize after a few years.

For more information:

1. Tobacco smoking and the risk of atrial fibrillation: https://journals.sagepub.com/doi/full/10.1177/2047487318780435

Exercise and Atrial Fibrillation

To begin with, if you plan to incorporate any kind of exercise, no matter how light it might seem, always keep your doctor informed and get their permission and advice. Depending on your AFib symptoms, your doctor might approve certain exercises to help you better control your AFib condition and avoid triggering episodes of AFib during exercise.

With AFib, exercise needs to be done at the right level to maximize gains and to mitigate risks. Exercise seems to improve just about any chronic condition including heart disease and AFib. But with a tricky condition like AFib, you may suffer symptoms that might worsen with exertion. Hence, you must tread a fine line to gain benefits without worsening your AFib.

There are several AFib symptoms that can make exercising more difficult and even risky. These can include:

- Dizziness
- Heart Palpitations
- Anxiety
- Excessive Sweating
- Shortness of Breath

AFib can potentially make exercising harder since AFib patients find that their heartbeat becomes faster and more painful with even moderate exertion. If your heartbeat becomes too fast, you may experience several symptoms including chest pain, shortness of breath, or dizziness.

Despite the risks, exercise can help AFib patients in many ways. Exercise brings down the risk of coronary artery disease which is a major risk factor for AFib development and progression. Exercise can also reduce your blood pressure and reduce your weight if you are overweight – both weight loss and improving high blood pressure are crucial long-term goals for AFib patients. Light, slow and gentle exercise can also possibly bring down your heart rate if done right. This will come as a major relief for AFib patients since they may sometimes face an unstable and painful heartbeat.

Exercise also helps to relieve stress and anxiety which can worsen AFib symptoms for many patients. The correct level of exercise can thus greatly improve the quality of life for AFib patients and bring down several risk factors.

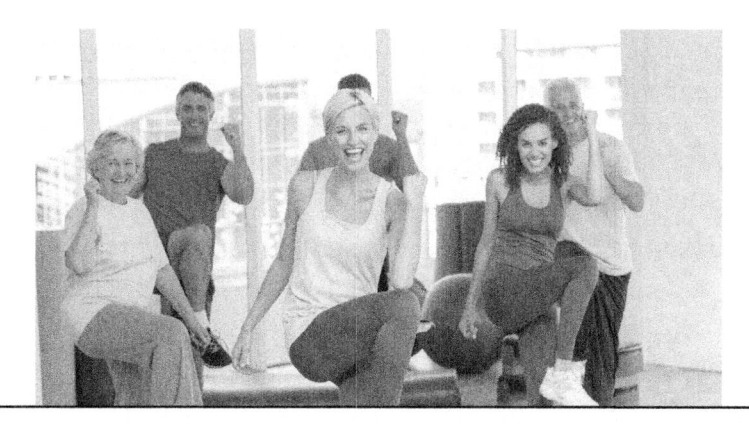

Exercise can be very beneficial and safe for most AFib patients.

One important safety point is to never exceed your limits. If exercise feels too uncomfortable or painful, then you must stop immediately and take a rest.

Another key point to be careful about is to do everything gradually. Don't hit top gear from the start. Instead, gently work your way up after starting with gentle stretching. Besides stretching, you should do low impact exercises like walking slowly for at least 10 minutes. You can then slowly and gradually increase the pace of your exercise to what your body can handle comfortably. For this, you will need to follow your doctor's advice as well as listen to your own body. Over time you may notice that you can significantly increase your exercise routine.

Drink plenty water before exercising; I frequently tell my AFib patients to pre-hydrate prior to exercise. The dehydration that can come from sweating and exercise can trigger an episode of AFib.

After doing warmups, you can exercise according to what your doctor has planned out for you or based on your own fitness level. If your health permits, you can go hiking or power walking without putting undue strain on your heart. You can do it outside to benefit from fresh air if possible. If not, you can also safely exercise indoors using a treadmill, an exercise bike or elliptical machine.

It is important for all beginners, no matter how young or healthy they are, to start gently and then to make their exercise regimen more challenging as they build strength, fitness and stamina. This reduces the possibility of injuries. This is even more important for AFib patients; it can take some time to build up the fitness level that you may desire. But do not let the time factor dishearten you because if you exercise regularly, your body will gradually adapt by becoming more fit.

At first, you might become exhausted by working out for just five minutes. This is not unusual if you have a sedentary lifestyle as many heart patients often do. After a few weeks, you might take it to 10 minutes before experiencing exhaustion. As you slowly become comfortable with your current exercise load, you can challenge yourself further in small increments amounting to a few minutes. You can keep raising the bar until you feel you are doing enough exercise as is necessary for your health.

High-impact and high-intensity exercise is not a good idea for anyone who is just beginning an exercise program. AFib patients, in particular, must begin with lighter exercises of short intervals to build up their fitness, and to reduce risks of exacerbating AFib during exercise. As your fitness increases, you can start adding some higher intensity workouts.

You should ideally avoid exercises that increase the risk of accidents, like outdoor biking and skiing. You should replace these exercises with ones that you can do safely with minimal risk of accident or injury. This is particularly important for AFib patients who are on blood-thinning medications since these medicines can increase the risk of uncontrolled bleeding.

After taking all the precautions as mentioned above, if you still undergo AFib attacks due to exercise, you should stop and inform your doctor or physical therapist about it. Your doctor might have you undergo treatment with specific medication to ensure that your heartbeat is not too fast or erratic during exercise. This may improve your chances of success with safe exercise. In addition, if you are experiencing chest pain with exercise, your doctor will likely want to evaluate you for coronary artery disease with a circulation test, such as a stress test.

Using a smart fitness watch with a heart rate tracker while doing exercise can be helpful for many patients with AFib. These devices are usually powered with an app that can give you detailed heartbeat statistics by connecting with your smartphone, computer or laptop.

There are several popular fitness trackers that consumers can purchase, like a Fitbit or Apple Watch, which both provide numerous models each having its own blend of features including heart rate monitoring capabilities.

The Centers for Disease Control and Prevention states that moderate physical activity should mean no more than 50 to 70 percent of your maximum heart rate. To follow this guideline, you can easily use a fitness device mentioned above.

Here is what you should know about your maximum heart rate:

To find out your maximum heart rate, deduct your age from 220. So, if you are 60 years of age for instance, your maximum heart rate will be 220 – 60 = 160 beats per minute.

For calculating the safe range of heartbeat for moderate exercise, you should find the upper limit and the lower limit. To find the upper limit, multiply the maximum heart rate by 0.7. In the example mentioned above, this will turn out to be 160 x 0.7 = 112 heartbeats per minute. The lower limit is found by multiplying the maximum heartbeat by 0.5. For the age of 60, this will turn out to be 160 x 0.5 = 80 beats per minute. Hence, if you are 60 years old, then the safe range of heartbeats for moderate exercise is between 80 and 112 beats per minute.

If you are taking pharmaceuticals called beta blockers, such as metoprolol, you may find that your heart rate is not increasing substantially even with moderate-intensity exercise. The reason for this is that beta blockers slow down your heart rate and bring down your blood pressure. So, even if you are working out at moderate intensity, your heart rate may not go up by much if you are on beta blockers.

It is all right to feel nervous about exercise if you have AFib. If you qualify, you may reduce your concerns by participating in a monitored cardiac rehabilitation program. Your doctor may prescribe this program before you start working out.

You must also be aware that certain AFib symptoms might be exacerbated with exercise. You might even start experiencing chest pain during exercise. You must stop exercising immediately if you undergo chest pain and take a rest. If the pain does not abate even with a short break, then you should call the local emergency number or 911.

There are other warning symptoms to look out for during exercise, including:

- Disorientation or confusion
- Shooting pain in the arm
- Shortness of breath that is not subsiding even with rest
- Trouble thinking clearly
- Slurred speech
- Unexpected weakness in part of your body
- Loss of consciousness

If you experience any other symptom that is painful or making you feel unwell during exercise, then you should call your doctor immediately or seek emergency medical treatment.

Sleep Apnea and AFib

Sleep apnea is a serious medical condition that affects 18 million people in the US and over 100 million people around the world. A staggering 85 percent of cases are not diagnosed at all. Several clinical studies have demonstrated that sleep apnea is frequently under-diagnosed in AFib patients.

Sleep apnea refers to very shallow breathing or complete cessation of breathing during sleep. The most common kind of sleep apnea is obstructive sleep apnea which happens due to blockage of the air passage by the tongue during sleep. Sleep apnea causes the victim to partially or fully wake up from sleep since they have trouble breathing. These incidents can happen numerous times during the night; as a result, sleep is heavily disrupted. People with sleep apnea may not even realize they are waking up several times during

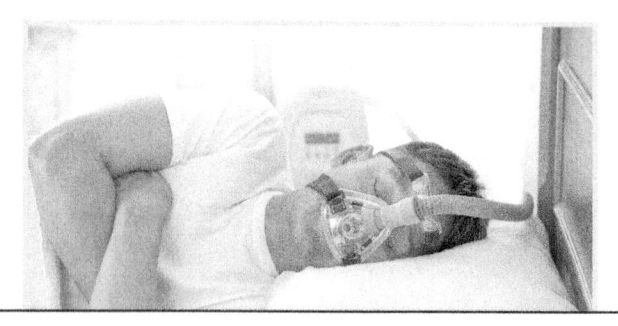

The most common treatment for sleep apnea is a CPAP mask.

sleep.

People with sleep apnea often snore loudly and wake up from sleep in a state of anxiety due to lack of oxygen. Since sleep is heavily disrupted, people with sleep apnea often feel drowsy, stressed, and lethargic during the day. Over the long term, sleep apnea can increase the risk for diabetes, accidents, high blood pressure, and heart disease including AFib.

Clinical studies have frequently demonstrated that sleep apnea can increase the risk for AFib. Around half of patients with AFib also suffer from sleep apnea. People with sleep apnea have a four times higher risk of developing AFib than people who don't have this condition. One reason why sleep apnea leads to a higher AFib risk is that sleep disruption plays a direct role in conditions like hypertension, weight gain, and fatigue, which are direct risk factors for the development of AFib.

Sleep apnea can also induce arrhythmias during sleep. The heart undergoes chemical changes and stress each time the person stops breathing and has decreased oxygen levels as a result. The adverse impact on the heart from oxygen deprivation may be a key reason why sleep apnea can lead to AFib.

Research also suggests that sleep apnea may make it more difficult to control AFib since it can possibly interfere with the effectiveness of AFib medications and treatment. AFib patients without sleep apnea often respond better to treatment than AFib patients with uncontrolled or untreated sleep apnea. AFib patients who have gone through catheter ablation procedures or cardioversion are more likely to have recurrent AFib episodes if they have untreated sleep apnea. Studies are increasingly showing that for people with both AFib and sleep apnea, overall treatment will be more successful if it addresses both AFib and sleep apnea simultaneously.

Considering the deleterious effects of sleep apnea on AFib, every patient with AFib should undergo testing for sleep apnea. You should also be tested for sleep apnea if you are gasping for air upon waking up, experiencing seriously disturbed sleep, feeling unusually drowsy and lethargic during the day, having headaches upon waking up, etc. In my opinion, every patient with atrial fibrillation should be screened for sleep apnea since they commonly occur together. In addition, proper treatment of sleep apnea can make a significant improvement in AFib symptoms and make treatment options for AFib more successful.

Treating sleep apnea is also a useful method of improving AFib symptoms. The CPAP oxygen mask is the most commonly recommended method for treating sleep apnea. By enhancing breathing at night, the CPAP oxygen mask can noticeably improve AFib symptoms in many patients. Treating AFib in conjunction with properly treated sleep apnea can also improve the success rate of procedures such as an ablation or cardioversion.

The CPAP mask works by helping you to breathe more consistently during the night while sleeping. However, many people complain that these masks are uncomfortable and make them feel claustrophobic. In case you are experiencing such problems, then you should try out different varieties of masks since CPAP masks are available in different shapes and sizes. There are nasal only masks besides the typical full-face masks. You should talk to your doctor to find out which configuration will work best for you.

These masks are important particularly for AFib patients with sleep apnea who find that they are suffering from AFib upon waking up at night. It is very possible that sleep apnea is to blame for a flare up of AFib at night. Hence, getting tested for sleep apnea and using a CPAP mask if necessary is critical for many AFib patients.

Currently, there are no proven supplements for treating sleep apnea. Besides a CPAP mask, you should cut out alcohol, avoid tobacco and maintain healthy weight since these factors influence the prevalence of sleep apnea as well. Besides controlling AFib symptoms, treating sleep apnea may also be beneficial for improving high blood pressure.

For More Information:

1. The Interplay between Obstructive Sleep Apnea and Atrial Fibrillation: https://www.ncbi.nlm.nih.gov/pmc/articles/PMC5732262/

2. Atrial Fibrillation and Obstructive Sleep Apnea: https://www.ahajournals.org/doi/10.1161/CIRCEP.117.005890

Does Stress Affect AFib Symptoms?

Stress can influence AFib since it can worsen several risk factors behind AFib. Heightened stress can raise the incidence of AFib attacks, and increase their severity and duration. Many AFib patients find they are suffering from more frequent AFib episodes during stressful times.

Stress influences and triggers AFib in a number of ways.

Stress increases blood pressure, which is a major risk factor for AFib. In addition, the habits people develop during periods of increased stress can also trigger episodes of AFib. Too much caffeine, alcohol abuse, and tobacco use can all worsen your stress and increase AFib symptoms. Stressful conditions also interfere with your sleep which can negatively impact AFib.

Removing all sources of stress may not exactly cure AFib. However, stress reduction can significantly reduce the severity, duration and frequency of AFib symptoms. Hence, stress management is a key component of AFib treatment for many people.

There are several avenues for reducing stress such as support groups, exercise, meditation, and yoga to name a few. Always discuss with your doctor which methods for stress reduction may be best for you.

In the Yoga My Heart Study, 52 patients were assigned to perform twice weekly structured yoga for three months. The investigators found that yoga training reduced symptomatic AFib episodes, improved high blood pressure, and improved depression and anxiety scores.

For More Information:

1. The Yoga My Heart Study: https://pubmed.ncbi.nlm.nih.gov/23375926/

The Truth Behind Weight Loss and Reversal of Atrial Fibrillation

Obesity is a serious health problem that can make you more vulnerable to multiple, dangerous medical conditions like heart disease, sleep apnea, diabetes and high blood pressure. Obesity is also a significant risk factor for AFib.

There are several ways in which obesity can increase your risk of getting Afib. As mentioned above, obesity predisposes you to dangerous, chronic conditions like heart diseases, sleep apnea, diabetes, high blood pressure and other chronic illnesses that are significant risk factors for AFib.

In addition, it has been noted that fat tissue located around the heart is chemically active and can increase local inflammation around the heart which can then lead to progression of AFib.

If you are obese but do not have the typical medical conditions associated with obesity, you should still be very careful since obesity can also increase the levels of inflammatory substances in your body. These inflammatory substances can eventually cause several medical conditions including AFib.

The standard advice for AFib patients for many years has been to lose weight if they are overweight. This advice was then validated by the 2015 Legacy Trial. During this study, researchers monitored over a thousand patients for more than five years. According to the results of this study, patients that lost more than 10 percent of their body mass saw a six-fold improvement with their AFib symptoms compared to controls. In fact, several patients who lost a substantial amount of weight had little to no AFib symptoms.

However, you must bear in mind that there are many considerations besides weight loss that may have a role to play in improving your AFib symptoms. But there is no doubt that overweight AFib patients often see a remarkable improvement in their symptoms after substantial weight loss. AFib patients should take heart that substantial weight loss can possibly mitigate several symptoms to the point that they are minimally noticeable. Even if these symptoms do not go away completely, there is a major improvement in the duration, frequency and severity of AFib symptoms.

Having discussed the remarkable benefits of weight loss for AFib patients, it needs no mention that it is easier said than done. But with determination, discipline and the right strategy it can be done even if it takes several months. Weight control is a key component of any long-term AFib treatment strategy.

If you would like my help to implement these lifestyle modifications in your life, including a step-by-step guide for improving nutrition and weight loss in an AFib focused manner, then consider my online program, Take Control Over AFib. In this structured online program, I will help you build a framework to implement many of the lifestyle modifications I discussed above, including weight loss, reducing inflammation, stress management, and sleep hygiene. In addition, this program has a focus on long-term results with the support to keep you motivated. Many of my students have noticed reduced AFib symptoms in as little as two weeks. In addition, many more students have been able to significantly reduce medications and improve symptoms several months after starting the program.

To learn more about the Take Control Over AFib program, visit https://www.takecontroloverafib.com

For More Information:

1. The Legacy Trial on Weight Loss and Atrial Fibrillation: https://www.onlinejacc.org/content/65/20/2159

What Are Common Treatment Options for Atrial Fibrillation?

Common Medical Therapy for AFib

Treatment options for AFib can include medications, nonsurgical catheter-based procedures and surgical procedures.

Medications are usually prescribed to reduce the risk of developing blood clots that can cause stroke. The majority of patients with AFib will be prescribed blood-thinning medications for stroke risk reduction. In addition, other pharmaceutical medications may be prescribed for controlling the rhythm of the heart as well as the heart rate.

Blood Thinning Medications for Stroke Risk Reduction

Blood thinning medications are frequently administered to prevent the formation of blood clots and also to treat an existing blood clot. The oldest blood thinning medication prescribed in this regard is warfarin. This medication was first approved in 1954 and for decades was the only approved blood thinning medication for atrial fibrillation. However, the FDA has approved direct acting oral anticoagulants over the last several years that may be safer and more effective then warfarin, like apixaban, edoxaban, rivaroxaban and dabigatran. As of the latest 2019 Atrial Fibrillation Treatment Guidelines Update, aspirin is no longer recommended as a blood thinner for atrial fibrillation. This is due to aspirin's relatively weak blood thinning effects and its minimal reduction in stroke risk.

Please see my previous discussion on stroke risk reduction with medications for further details on blood thinning medications. In this previous section I thoroughly discuss benefits and risks of blood thinning medications.

Heart Rate Controlling Medications

There are also several heart rate controlling medications commonly prescribed for AFib patients.

Beta Blockers are one of the most commonly prescribed medications for AFib. These medications work by slowing down your heartbeat. Many AFib patients find relief and feel better when their heart rate comes under control. Beta blockers commonly used may include:

- Timolol
- Propranolol
- Nadolol
- Metoprolol
- Carvedilol
- Bisoprolol
- Atenolol

Calcium channel blockers are another type of heart rate controlling medications commonly used for AFib. They can also slow down the heart rate in AFib patients and they can also reduce the strength of contractions. The most commonly used calcium channel blockers for AFib include verapamil and dilitiazem.

Digoxin is another commonly used medication that works by slowing down the rate at which electrical current is conducted to the ventricle (lower chambers of the heart) from the atria. Digoxin has been available for well over 50 years and is commonly used for atrial fibrillation. One benefit of digoxin over beta blockers and calcium channel blockers is the fact that it does not typically lower blood pressure. This makes it an attractive option for heart rate control when the patient's blood pressure is low.

However, digoxin can have significant side effects and risks as well. Elderly patients and those with abnormal kidney function may develop toxic levels of this medication. Recent studies have even shown that patients prescribed digoxin with an elevated digoxin level have an increased risk of death. So even though it is a medication that is used commonly, it still needs to be monitored very carefully and drug levels should be check with a blood test on occasion.

Heart Rhythm Controlling Medications

Heart rhythm controlling medications try to bring your heart rhythm back to normal. This process is known as a pharmacological or chemical cardioversion. These medications can also be very potent to prevent episodes of atrial fibrillation, more potent than traditional beta blockers. However, many of these medications have the potential to cause serious side effects and need to be monitored closely and used in the correct patient.

Sodium channel blockers slow down the ability of the heart to conduct rapid electricity in order to restore optimal heart rhythm. Quinidine, propafenone and flecainide are some examples of commonly used sodium channel blockers. I use flecainide and propafenone very commonly in my AFib patients. I feel that they are safe long-term medications to use when monitored closely and used in the correct patients. For example, these types of medications should not be used in patients with underlying coronary artery disease or congestive heart failure. Especially in patients with coronary artery disease, previous studies have linked these medications with an increased risk for dangerous ventricular arrhythmias. As a result, I usually perform coronary artery disease screening in patients before I begin to use these medications. In addition, I perform routine follow-up screening for coronary artery disease, such as with a stress test, every two years for patients on these medications.

Potassium channel blockers try to restore the heart's natural rhythm by reducing electrical currents from potassium channels in the heart that can lead to AFib. Examples of potassium channel blockers include dofetilide, sotalol, dronedarone (brand name of

Multaq), and amiodarone. These are also medications that I have commonly used in patients with AFib. However, there are again restrictions on these medications to be aware of. The most serious risk of all these medications is called QT prolongation. This is the time it takes for the heartbeat to reset, when it is significantly prolonged it can also increase the risk for dangerous ventricular arrhythmias. Dofetilide and sotalol are both cleared by the kidneys, so patients with abnormal kidney function will have an increased risk for dangerous side effects from these medications.

Special note should be made of amiodarone since it is likely the most commonly used of all these heart rhythm controlling medications. It is statistically the strongest medication to control or prevent atrial fibrillation. It is available in both intravenous and pill form. One of the benefits of amiodarone is that it typically works rapidly and does not usually affect blood pressure. Thus, it is a common treatment of choice for patients in a hospital or emergency room since it rapidly improves atrial fibrillation with little effect on the blood pressure. It is overall rare to see side effects from amiodarone during short-term use such as in a hospital setting.

However, of all the medications for heart rhythm control, amiodarone has the longest list of long-term use side effects. There are a wide variety of side effects from the medication which may be irreversible. Long-term usage of amiodarone can cause lung, liver, and thyroid toxicity. It can also significantly impair vision and cause nerve damage. Although I frequently use amiodarone in my patients as a short-term plan, I usually discontinue the medication within six months to avoid the long-term toxicities of this medication.

Cardioversion for AFib

An electrical cardioversion is a type of medical procedure for the treatment of rapid and abnormal heart rhythms like AFib. A cardioversion is a common procedure used for atrial fibrillation and usually takes only a few minutes to perform. During the cardioversion process, an electrical current applied to the chest wall can help to restore the heart rhythm to the normal sinus rhythm.

A cardioversion is somewhat similar to when someone gets their heart shocked on television, only a lot less dramatic. We do give a "CLEAR!" order to let everyone in the room know the cardioversion shock is about to happen, so television did get something correct.

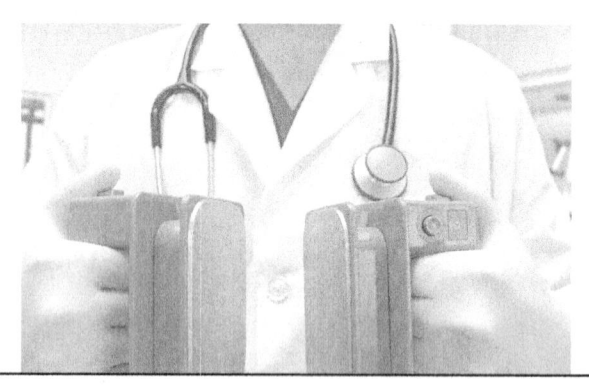

A cardioversion is typically not as dramatic as it appears on television.

Understanding the heart's conduction system is imperative for understanding how cardioversion works. The heart is composed mainly of muscle tissue. The heart is divided into four chambers. The upper chambers are known as the atria while the lower chambers are called the ventricles. Each chamber has a valve so that blood can flow in the right direction.

Heart muscles contract from electrical impulses. When the heart rhythm is normal, each electrical pulse is transferred in the correct way over nerves and heart muscle to the ventricles from the atria. Specialized pacemaker cells known as the sinus node generate the electrical impulses in the atria under normal conditions. These cells are situated in the top of the right atrium.

When the impulse leaves the sinus node, it goes on to activate the atria. The electrical impulse then moves along special heart fibers that transfer the electrical impulse to the ventricle resulting in a contraction, or heartbeat. All muscle cells in the ventricles are activated during the contraction. A normal heart rhythm requires electrical current conduction and muscle contraction in the correct order. If this order is disturbed, then the result is an abnormal heart pattern also known as arrhythmia.

In any rapid cardiac arrhythmia, an abnormally quick electrical process overrides the sinus node function. There are several kinds of rapid cardiac arrhythmias, including AFib.

In a healthy heart rhythm, an electrical impulse travels from the top of the heart to the bottom after which it dissipates. The next consecutive electrical impulse starts in the sinus node independently.

In some cases, heart tissue can make a short circuit or an electrical loop. If an electrical current comes into such a loop, then under certain circumstances it will go through the loop indefinitely, over and over again. It's like driving on a circle shaped road over, and over again.

In addition, multiple of these abnormal electrical reentrant loops can form under certain circumstances which can lead to chaotic and rapid arrhythmias that include atrial fibrillation.

In a cardioversion, a high energy shock is delivered towards the heart muscle from the chest wall. As a result of this high energy shock, all the conduction tissue and cardiac muscle tissue are simultaneously activated and reset. This can disrupt the reentrant circuit thus putting a stop to the indefinitely repeating electrical impulse. This can stop most arrhythmias. If the reentrant circuit is disrupted and the arrhythmia halts, then the sinus node can start firing once again restoring normal heart rhythm. The normal sinus node will almost always restart when the abnormal circuit is stopped with a cardioversion.

A cardioversion procedure is usually carried out in a special room for medical procedures that has the necessary equipment for monitoring oxygen levels, respiratory rate, blood pressure, heart rate and of course, heart rhythm.

The high energy electrical shock is too painful for patients who are awake. Hence patients undergoing the procedure are first sedated through an intravenous medication. Patients often do not remember what went on during the procedure.

The skin is shaved if necessary and electrode paddles or patches are brought into contact with the skin's surface. One patch is placed on the right upper chest while the other one is applied below the shoulder blade, the back or the lower left chest. After the patient is sedated, an electrical current is transmitted through the patches. While most of the current is absorbed by the chest wall, some of it reaches the heart muscles. The energy level applied for the shock depends on the type of arrhythmia and the patient's body habitus. Patient's that are significantly obese typically require higher energy during a cardioversion, since more energy is needed to get through the chest wall and reach the heart. If the first shock fails to deliver the right results, then a second shock may be applied to restore normal heart rhythm. If required, shocks with higher energy may also be applied.

The cardioversion itself usually only takes a few seconds. Sedating the patient takes a longer time. The patient is monitored for usually around 60 minutes following the procedure after the anesthetic medications wear off.

The patient can typically leave the hospital a few hours following the procedure if their condition is stable. They will be closely monitored during this time. Patients who are sedated should not drive before 24 hours have elapsed. A relative or friend should drive them home.

A cardioversion is used for several kinds of arrhythmias; it is particularly useful for atrial fibrillation with an overall good success rate. However, there are conditions where the success rate may be lower, for instance if the atrium is enlarged or if the atrial fibrillation has gone untreated for a long time. In addition, even though a cardioversion is frequently successful at that moment, it does not mean that AFib cannot come back, sometimes as soon as the following day. This is why it is important to take your medications even after a cardioversion to reduce the risk of recurrence of AFib.

There are some small risks associated with cardioversion. If a blood clot exists, it might break loose due to the procedure and result in thromboembolism or stroke. Hence, to counter this threat, the patient is usually prescribed warfarin or another blood thinner a few at least a few weeks before and after the procedure. For patients that are not on a blood thinner prior to a cardioversion, a procedure called a transesophageal echo can performed to check for a blood clot in the heart prior to the cardioversion. While a patient is sedated a probe about the size of a finger is inserted through the mouth into the esophagus. The doctor is then able to take thorough images of the heart to exclude the presence of a blood clot. Usually, if needed, the transesophageal echo and cardioversion can be performed in the same procedure.

In my experience, a cardioversion is successful about 90 percent of the time to stop AFib and restore sinus rhythm. But performing a cardioversion is only half of the battle; keeping someone in normal rhythm is the other part of the battle. I frequently give the example of a cell phone or computer, if it is not working properly, it is usually helpful to restart the device. However, if there is an underlying problem, then the same issue will continue to happen again.

The same thing can happen with AFib, that despite a successful cardioversion, atrial fibrillation can recur due to an underlying problem. There are many ways that you can reduce the recurrence of AFib after a cardioversion, including medical therapy, lifestyle modifications, treating sleep apnea if present, or in some cases - an invasive procedure like a catheter ablation which I will discuss in the next section.

But what happens if a cardioversion does not work? What options do patients have when they experience an unsuccessful cardioversion? The first option would be to do nothing. In some cases, the patient may not be a candidate for alternative treatment options. In these cases, patients will remain in atrial fibrillation and remain on medical therapy. A second option would be to repeat the cardioversion in a few weeks after an adjustment of medical therapy. I have had several cases where adjustments of medications resulted in a successful cardioversion a few weeks after a failed one. Most of the time, medication adjustments involve strong anti-arrhythmic medications like amiodarone.

The last option if a cardioversion does not work would be an ablation procedure discussed in the next section. An ablation procedure is a much more aggressive option then a cardioversion, so not everyone will be a candidate for this option.

Ablation Procedures for AFib

An ablation procedure treats an arrhythmia (an irregular or fast heart rhythm) by intentionally scarring heart tissue in order to disrupt the erratic electrical impulses that are causing the arrhythmia. Unlike the natural scarring that happens due to AFib and its risk factors, an ablation procedure produces strategic scarring meant to reduce atrial fibrillation. I frequently tell patients the scar tissue created during an ablation procedure is like creating an electrical roadblock to block the misfires of AFib and allow the normal rhythm to take control again.

Your doctor may recommend this treatment if medications or lifestyle modifications are not providing sufficient results for your AFib symptoms, especially if your symptoms are getting worse despite standard medications. Usually, an ablation procedure is not the first line choice for treating AFib due to inherent risks for any invasive procedure.

If your AFib symptoms are becoming worse despite medications, your doctor may recommend an ablation procedure to stop symptoms from deteriorating. After this procedure, patients often report an improvement in AFib symptoms.

There are three kinds of ablation procedures performed for atrial fibrillation:

1. Traditional Catheter Ablation for AFib

2. Surgical AFib Ablation Procedure

3. AV Node Ablation

Traditional Catheter Ablation for AFib

The most common ablation procedure performed on AFib patients is a traditional catheter ablation, where the main goal is pulmonary vein isolation. I will further discuss the procedure in detail below. If you have agreed with your doctor to proceed with a catheter ablation, what are the next typical steps?

The next typical step is to make sure you are medically optimized as best as possible prior to the procedure. This may include steps such as adjusting blood pressure medications or treating any congestive heart failure symptoms, for example. Preoperative testing would likely include blood work, which would test items such as your blood counts and kidney function. Likely there may be a pre-procedure chest X-ray ordered, which is used as a baseline and can be compared post procedure to another X-ray if needed. Your doctor may also get a pre-procedure cardiac CT or MRI; these may be used to better identify the anatomy of your heart, such as the size of the left atrium, evaluate for a presence or absence of a blood clot in your heart prior to the procedure, and sometimes these images can also be used to assess for scar tissue in your atrium.

Alternatively, your doctor may schedule a transesophageal echo (also called a TEE) either the morning of the procedure or the day prior to the procedure. This a very detailed ultrasound of your heart usually used to evaluate for a presence or absence of a blood clot in your heart prior to the procedure. All of this information can be useful to your doctor to develop a strategy for your ablation procedure.

In the morning of the procedure, you will likely be prepared in a pre-procedure area. Typically, an IV is inserted to give medications during the procedure. You will likely be shaved along your groin (this is where your doctor typically enters your veins for the procedure), also your chest may be shaved if needed as multiple cardiac electrodes are placed on the chest during the procedure to monitor your heartbeat very closely. During the pre-procedure you will also likely meet your anesthesiologist. Most ablation procedures are done with anesthesia, as the process of burning or freezing inside of your heart can be painful for someone who is awake.

Now, what actually happens when the patient goes to sleep? During the procedure you will be lying on an X-ray table. The procedure begins with your doctor entering through the veins in your groin with a needle puncture, these veins are also called the femoral veins. Typically, multiple punctures are needed as there are multiple catheters used during the procedure. Your doctor will then advance the catheters into your heart. In order to perform an ablation for atrial fibrillation, your doctor will need to get into the left atrium, which is the left upper chamber of the heart; this is where most people's atrial fibrillation comes from. In order to get there, your doctor will typically need to do what is called a trans-septal puncture. Basically, your doctor will create a very small hole to cross from the right upper chamber to left upper chamber of your heart. This small hole usually heals on its own several weeks after the procedure. It sounds dramatic to describe that your doctor will intentionally create a small hole in your heart, but with proper safety equipment, this is a very routine part of the procedure that only takes a few minutes.

Once your doctor has all the necessary equipment in place, then he or she will start the ablation process. During an ablation for atrial fibrillation the most common targets are the pulmonary veins, located in the left atrium. Typically, patients have four pulmonary veins that drain blood from the lungs back to the heart. These pulmonary veins have extensions of nerves and heart tissue that can trigger episodes of atrial fibrillation. This is a common source for most patient's atrial fibrillation. As a result, the main goal during most ablation procedures for AFib is to make a strategic scar inside your heart to block these triggers around the pulmonary veins that can lead to episodes of atrial fibrillation. This scar does not affect the blood flow from the lungs back to your heart but does block those trigger areas to reduce your atrial fibrillation.

You doctor will likely ablate the tissue near the pulmonary veins using either radiofrequency (burning methods) or cryotherapy (freezing methods). The goal is to have a thorough ablation performed of all four pulmonary veins during the procedure. This is a process that can typically take around three hours to do. After completion of the pulmonary vein ablation, your doctor may do additional testing to see if you can still be induced into atrial fibrillation or another arrhythmia. What I tell patients is that this is the part that is customized per patient. Atrial fibrillation affects hearts in different ways, while inside of your heart your doctor can have a detailed assessment of how much atrial fibrillation has affected your heart, most commonly this is seen through the amount of scar tissue noted in your left atrium or by identifying additional triggers for atrial fibrillation which can be identified by giving a stimulant type medication during the procedure.

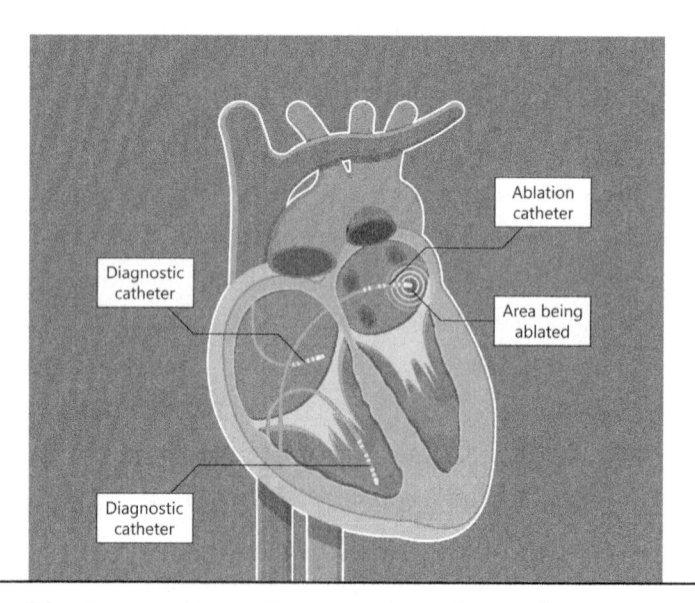

The ablation catheter is targeting the pulmonary veins in the left atrium during an ablation procedure.

After the procedure you will typically be transferred to a recovery area. Here your heartbeat and blood pressure will be monitored closely after the procedure. I typically order a chest X-ray after the procedure to make a comparison to the pre-procedure chest X-ray. I do this to check for signs of fluid accumulation in your lungs during the procedure which can later cause shortness of breath. It's not uncommon to have several liters of intravenous fluid given during a catheter ablation through both your anesthesiologist as well as with the ablation catheter itself. You will usually have to rest in bed for several hours, typically about four to six hours, to minimize risk of bleeding at your groin puncture site. Depending on your doctor's preference and your co-morbid medical conditions, some patients may be able to go home the same day, while some may need to stay overnight in the hospital to recover.

After the procedure you can except to have some groin bruising and soreness. However, you should never have severe pain in your groin or bleeding; if you have those please alert your doctor. Chest discomfort can also be expected due to the ablation process. The pain is due to inflammation from the procedure. It is typically a very positional discomfort, for example you may notice it more lying down versus sitting up. Again, it should not be severe pain; if you have severe pain please alert your doctor. For most patients these symptoms subside in a few days, but for some patients it can take over a week to fully recover from an ablation procedure.

But what about your atrial fibrillation? Do you get immediate relief after the procedure? Can you immediately stop medications after the ablation? Not so fast, unfortunately. I usually explain to patients that during an ablation you are making a strategic scar inside of your heart. Just like when you cut your skin, it does not heal or form a scar right away; there is a period of healing and waiting for the inflammation from the ablation procedure to subside. Because of this I typically wait for at least one month before I start to decrease medications for atrial fibrillation.

The long-term success rate of a catheter ablation in the treatment of AFib varies depending on the type and duration of AFib (i.e., paroxysmal vs persistent AFib) and previous structural remodeling of the heart. In general, the success rate usually ranges from 60-80 percent over one to two years of follow-up. Patients with paroxysmal atrial fibrillation have much higher success rates. On the other hand, patients that have more advanced stages of atrial fibrillation, such as persistent atrial fibrillation, are much more likely to need more than one procedure to get good control over atrial fibrillation.

As with any invasive procedure, please note that there are, of course, potential risks involved with a catheter ablation for AFib. In my experience, patients that are older, or that have a weakening of the heart muscle, called CHF, have higher risks for complications from an AFib ablation.

Here are some of the risks of atrial fibrillation ablation:

- Blood vessel damage

- Infection or bleeding where catheters were applied

- Damage to the electrical system of your heart. This may worsen AFib and a pacemaker will be needed to correct it.

- Heart valve damage

- Puncturing of heart tissue

- Pulmonary vein stenosis – veins between the lungs and heart become narrower

- Venous thromboembolism – blood clots form in lungs or legs

- Death (rare)

There are always precautions to take to minimize risks during any procedure. Optimizing additional health conditions such as high blood pressure, congestive heart failure, or chronic lung disease is essential for preoperative risk assessment. Your doctor will need to address your overall health condition to minimize the risks from an ablation procedure.

For More Information:

1. Animation on traditional catheter ablation for AFib: https://www.youtube.com/watch?v=SZ_ulfj-hIQ&t=162s

2. Animation on traditional ablation using a freezing balloon catheter: https://www.youtube.com/watch?v=jk9dEoqscnI

Surgical Ablation Procedures

There are many ways to perform an ablation procedure for AFib different from the traditional catheter ablation procedures discussed above. Another option for an ablation procedure is a surgical ablation procedure. The most common surgical ablation procedure performed is called a mini maze procedure. Overall, surgical ablation procedures are more aggressive, and with higher risks than a traditional catheter ablation procedure. As a result, not everyone with AFib is a good candidate for a surgical ablation procedure.

The Mini Maze Procedure

A cardiothoracic surgeon usually performs the mini maze procedure. It requires a few hours and does not usually require big incisions like traditional open heart surgery. Hence, the recovery time is shorter than a typical open heart surgery and most patients find an improvement in their AFib symptoms. However, patients will still likely stay in the hospital for a few days and may require several weeks to recover from a mini maze procedure.

In a mini maze procedure, the surgeon will access your heart through small incisions on both sides of the chest. Through these incisions, the surgeon will direct a thoracoscope, an ablation device and other surgical instruments. The thoracoscope is also called an endoscope. It is a camera that provides clear sight of the heart and blood vessels.

An energy source (usually burning energy or radiofrequency, sometimes cryotherapy) is then used for the procedure for the creation of the strategic scar tissue to create a conduction block that prevents irregular electrical pulses from disrupting the normal heart rhythm and to isolate pulmonary veins. In both a surgical ablation and a catheter-based ablation, pulmonary vein isolation is a goal of the procedure. In a mini maze, the surgeon also typically treats nerve bundles and the ligament of Marshall, areas of the heart that are collectively known as the ganglionic plexi. These nerves can also affect the severity of AFib and performing ablation on these nerves may reduce AFib. The surgeon will also typically clamp off or remove the left atrial appendage so that the risk of stroke and blood clots is usually reduced.

For patients with more advanced AFib symptoms (including both persistent and longstanding persistent AFib), newer techniques have made better outcomes possible. Additional ablation lesions are also frequently made at the bottom and the top of the atria and also other places like the mitral annulus which is an area near the mitral valve. Better procedures and tools have enhanced ablation effectiveness for areas of the heart that were previously hard to access and difficult to treat.

For paroxysmal atrial fibrillation, the reported success rate for the mini maze procedure stands between 80 to 90 percent. For more advanced stages of AFib, such as persistent and longstanding persistent AFib, the success rate of the mini maze ranges from 50 to 75 percent. There may be variations in the success rate depending on the energy source deployed. Developments in lesion sets and energy sources have improved the success rate of the mini maze in particular for persistent and the longstanding persistent varieties of AFib.

Some small studies have reported a higher success rate with surgical ablations like a mini maze versus a typical catheter ablation. However, patients undergoing a surgical ablation procedure typically stay in the hospital for several days post procedure with a longer recovery time when compared to a catheter ablation procedure. Overall, a surgical ablation procedure has higher risks compared to catheter ablation; some studies have noted complication rates of over 20 percent for surgical ablations.

As compared with a catheter ablation where there is a small risk of strokes and blood clots, with the mini maze, blood clots or procedural strokes are rarely noted since the procedure does not involve catheters inside of the heart.

However, there are still significant risks associated with any surgical ablation procedure. The following risks are associated with the mini maze procedure:

- Heart or blood vessel damage
- Pericarditis (heart inflammation)
- Phlebitis (vein inflammation)
- Collapsed lung. This can be corrected by means of a chest tube.

In general, some of the best candidates for a surgical ablation procedure are patients with a history of AFib who require open heart surgery for other reasons. For patients who have a history of AFib, who also require a coronary bypass surgery or valve surgery, such as a mitral valve surgery, I frequently recommend a mini maze or other surgical ablation procedure during the time of open heart surgery. In addition, the closure of the left atrial appendage during open heart surgery can significantly reduce long-term stroke risk.

However, as a stand-alone procedure, I would usually recommend to patients to attempt a traditional catheter ablation procedure over a surgical ablation procedure as a first measure. This is especially true for patients with earlier stages of AFib, such as paroxysmal atrial fibrillation. For paroxysmal atrial fibrillation, a catheter-based procedure has a comparable success rate to a surgical ablation procedure, and a much lower risk profile and much faster recovery time.

For patients with more advanced atrial fibrillation, such as persistent or long-standing persistent AFib, a surgical ablation may offer a higher success rate than a catheter-based ablation. However, this may come at a cost of a higher risk profile compared to a catheter ablation. Also, many patients with AFib may also have multiple health conditions in addition to Afib, thus making a surgical ablation too risky for some patients.

For More Information:

1. Video with further information on the mini maze procedure: https://www.youtube.com/watch?v=EVk1FrmuE7Q

The Hybrid or Convergent Procedure

The newest type of surgical ablation is called the Hybrid or Convergent procedure. In this hybrid approach the surgeon works on the outside of the heart and the EP performs an ablation on the inside of the heart in an attempt to create more thorough ablation lesions. In a small study of 27 patients, most of whom had long-standing persistent A-Fib, at six months 72.2 percent of patients were in sinus rhythm. Also, recent analysis of several studies has shown that the hybrid procedure may be more effective than a traditional catheter ablation but still with increased risks when compared to a traditional catheter ablation procedure, despite a minimally invasive approach when compared to a typical mini maze procedure.

Overall, I feel that the hybrid procedure has potential, but at this time there is not enough clinical trial data for me to recommend it to my patients. It may be an option to consider for patients with more advanced persistent AFib, or patients who have had a recurrence of AFib despite a traditional catheter ablation procedure.

For More Information:

1. The Convergent Procedure: https://www.youtube.com/watch?v=-LbEP17ncC8

The AV Node Ablation

Another type of ablation performed to treat AFib is an AV node ablation. An AV Node ablation is when you burn in the middle portion of the heart, where the electrical impulses of the upper and lower chamber of the heart connect, basically just to control the heart rate. The patient is still in AFib, but the heart rate is no longer capable of going too fast. The heart rate actually ends up going very slow after an AV node ablation. Because your heart rate goes very slow with this type of ablation, it's required to do it with a pacemaker, or in a patient who already has a pacemaker. This type of ablation is relatively simple to perform as a procedure and is a safer option for people with many additional health conditions who are deemed too frail or too sick for other types of ablation procedures.

However, I frequently tell patients that this type of ablation means that we have reached the end of the road. There is no going back after this ablation procedure. After an AV node ablation, the heart is permanently very slow, and the patient will depend on a pacemaker for the rest of his or her life.

An AV node ablation does not reverse or prevent AFib, it is simply a means to control the heart rate so that someone has a nice steady heartbeat with fewer medications. However, the patient will still remain in atrial fibrillation and will still likely require blood-thinning medications for stroke risk reduction.

With that said, I have had many patients that have done very well after an AV node ablation. So, in the right settings, in can be beneficial treatment strategy for several patients.

How Are Pacemakers Used for the Treatment of AFib?

When I meet with a patient to discuss treatment options about atrial fibrillation, I frequently get asked questions about pacemakers and how they can help with the management of atrial fibrillation. First, when I get this question from patients, I feel that patients are assuming that the pacemaker is going or cure atrial fibrillation. The first thing I want to say is that a pacemaker does not cure atrial fibrillation. But a pacemaker can certainly help in the management of atrial fibrillation in several situations.

1. Sick Sinus Syndrome

The first situation in which a pacemaker can help is when the atrial fibrillation just goes too slow either all the time or intermittently. There are circumstances where the pulse can go too slow or even pause. The pulse that you check when you're checking your heart rate comes from the bottom portion of the heart, or the ventricles. Even when a person is in atrial fibrillation, sometimes the bottom portion of the heart, or the pulse, can go too slow, or sometimes even pause. In some cases, the heart may be slow all the time. In these cases, a pacemaker can help with that intermittent or continuous slowness or pauses, especially if the slow heart rates are causing symptoms such as dizziness or fatigue.

2. Tachy-Brady Syndrome

A second circumstance in which a pacemaker can help is what's called tachy-brady syndrome. What that basically means is that when you are in AFib, your heart rate is going very fast, and you need fairly aggressive medication to help control the speed of the heart rate. However, when AFib stops and you go back into normal rhythm, your natural heartbeat is very slow. It can be very difficult to treat AFib when you have a fast heartbeat while in AFIb, and a very slow heartbeat when you're in normal rhythm.

In addition, when you're taking medications for rapid atrial fibrillation, your natural heartbeat may become suddenly very slow when AFib stops. People can then feel dizzy or lightheaded, sometimes patients may even pass out. In these situations, a pacemaker can help balance out the heart rate so that your natural heart rate is not too slow, and then when you are in AFiB, you can better tolerate medications so that your heart rate is not going so fast during AFib episodes. A pacemaker is a very useful treatment option for many patients with alternating fast and slow heart rates, especially if you're not a good candidate for more aggressive options like a catheter ablation procedure.

3. AV Node Ablation

The third way in which a pacemaker can help is combined with a simple type of ablation called an AV node ablation, which I discussed previously. An AV node ablation is when you burn in the middle portion of the heart, where the electrical impulses of the upper and lower chamber of the heart connect, basically just to control the heart rate. The patient is still in AFib, but the heart rate is no longer capable of going too fast. It actually ends up going very slow after an AV node ablation. Because your heart rate goes very slow with this type of ablation, it's required to do it with a pacemaker, or with a patient who already has a pacemaker.

In addition, there are a few extra features of a pacemaker which can be beneficial for patients with atrial fibrillation. A pacemaker is a very accurate way to record or document episodes of AFib. As a result, when your doctor checks your pacemaker, he or she will know exactly how many atrial fibrillation episodes you are having. The pacemaker will clearly document every episode of atrial fibrillation, listing the date, time, duration, and average heart rate for every AFib episode. Also, most pacemakers have a remote monitoring feature, which gives your doctor frequent summary reports, usually every three months as a routine. Many pacemakers can provide alerts much sooner than three months if needed as well. This feature can help notify your doctor of a significant increase in AFib episodes, for example. There have been numerous patients I have had to call in for an urgent appointment because of an abnormal home monitoring report. Lastly, there are an increasing number of features some pacemakers have to try to smooth out a heart rate and actively reduce the number of AFib episodes.

Natural Treatments for Atrial Fibrillation

In addition to the conventional treatments that your doctor prescribes, you can consider natural methods to further minimize the risk of AFib progression and to reduce symptoms. While these natural methods can help, they are in no way an alternative to what your doctor recommends. Always discuss with your doctor about any natural method that you wish to adopt for your treatment.

When most people think of natural treatment, they are typically assuming that they can take a natural supplement that will treat or reverse atrial fibrillation. However, real natural treatment, that has been studied and proven to be beneficial in atrial fibrillation patients, involves lifestyle modifications and commitment.

There has been an abundance of scientific studies that show lifestyle modifications and weight loss can improve and potentially reverse atrial fibrillation. Multiple studies have shown that nutritional changes, weight loss, and reducing inflammation can have a dramatic improvement in AFib symptoms, and these methods have been studied in thousands of AFib patients. In addition, there are also multiple clinical studies that support improvement in atrial fibrillation symptoms with treatment for anxiety and stress, reducing alcohol intake, and improving sleep and sleep related disorders such as sleep apnea, just to name a few.

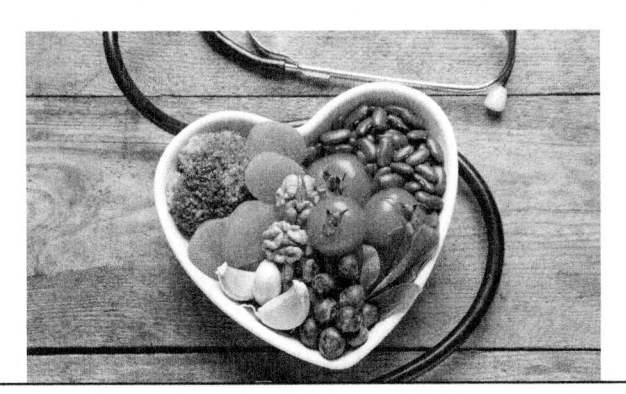

Following a heart healthy diet can lead to tremendous improvements in AFib Symptoms.

Following a heart friendly diet can help you with AFib. You will need to consume a diet that is rich in fiber and nutrients. Thus, your diet must include whole grains, beans, fruits and vegetables. When you consider whole grain items, you should consider real whole grains like oats, quinoa, or brown rice. Minimize red meat and use lean protein in its place, especially fatty fish. I frequently tell my patients, "try to keep your food as close as possible to how it came from the ground or an animal." Some of the biggest culprits for weight gain and inflammation are foods that have been processed from the original product.

Besides eating healthy foods, you should also take care to limit the consumption of inflammatory foods that can possibly worsen AFib. The following inflammatory foods I previously discussed in more detail when I discussed food triggers for AFib. I emphasis again the importance of minimizing or completely eliminating the foods below:

- High Sodium Foods
- Refined Carbohydrates
- MSG
- Trans Fats
- Saturated Fats
- Alcohol
- Aspartame
- Casein and Gluten (especially if you are allergic to these)

Besides participating in regular exercise, you should also make sure that you get enough sleep. Good quality sleep can help you recover from your workout and reduce the risk of several diseases. There has also been a clear association with fatigue and poor sleep hygiene and worsening of AFib symptoms.

You can also try out stress busting techniques like gentle stretching, deep breathing, mindfulness, and yoga. Remaining socially active can also help you to avoid stress.

Special Circumstances

Patients With Both Atrial Fibrillation and Coronary Artery Disease

Coronary artery disease and AFib are some of the most common medical conditions related to the heart. Coronary artery disease or CAD is the most common type of cardiovascular disease and atrial fibrillation is the most common heart arrhythmia. If you have both, then you need to know about the special precautions for managing both of these heart conditions.

Coronary artery disease is the biggest killer of men and women in the United States. This is the kind of cardiovascular disease that most people know about since it happens through the narrowing and hardening of arteries and can lead to heart attacks. In coronary artery disease, plaque and cholesterol build up on the interior of arteries. With the passage of time, heart muscles can weaken from coronary artery disease and significantly raise the risk of heart attacks, arrhythmias and chest pain.

To better understand both illnesses you must know what sets them apart. AFib happens because of irregular heartbeat while CAD is due to plaque buildup in the arteries. While AFib is frequently considered an electrical disorder of the heart, CAD is usually considered a plumbing related disorder of the heart. Hence, the two conditions are quite distinct even though they share common risk factors and symptoms. It is still possible to have AFib even if your coronary arteries are clear.

AFib and CAD both have similar common risk factors in the form of smoking, obesity, sleep apnea, diabetes, hypertension and alcohol. Inflammation plays a key role in both conditions and can accelerate their progression if not controlled. Since these conditions are so common and closely related, it is advisable to get tested for both if you have one of these conditions. Hence, AFib patients should get tested for CAD at appropriate intervals to catch the disease in its early stages before it does any significant damage.

Although both AFib and coronary artery disease are similar and closely related, having one does not mean that you are guaranteed the other. Hence, if you have AFib, it does not necessarily imply that you will have CAD. It does, however, mean that the risk of getting CAD is higher in patients with AFib.

If you first develop coronary artery disease and are then diagnosed with AFib, then your AFib treatment will have to factor in your CAD treatment, especially if you have a past history of stents or coronary bypass surgery. With CAD, your AFib treatment plan may differ from the treatment plan for an AFib patient without CAD.

Beta blockers are commonly used for the treatment of AFib. Carvedilol, propranolol, and metoprolol are some of the drugs commonly used for helping to slow down an overly fast heart rate which is quite common in AFib patients. Beta blockers are commonly used for both AFib and coronary artery disease. Antiarrhythmics are stronger medications that have a bigger impact on the heart rate, which can be beneficial for many AFib patients. If you have CAD or have undergone coronary bypass surgery, then you face a higher risk of complications from antiarrhythmics. The increased risk of side effects from some powerful antiarrhythmic drugs makes them unsuitable for many people with CAD and those who have had bypass surgery.

If you have AFib and a stent, then you may need two or more blood thinning medications to reduce the risk of clotting from both these factors. As you would imagine, the use of multiple blood thinners will increase the risk of bleeding side effects. However, there are typically not many options besides the use of multiple anticoagulants if you are an AFib patient with a coronary artery stent.

People with stents in their hearts need blood-thinning medications like Brilinta, Plavix, Effient or Aspirin. These medications can keep your stent open, but they work different by impacting platelets, which are tiny cells that allow blood clotting. These medications work by blocking platelets to thin your blood. These drugs are effective for keeping your stent open, but they do not work as well for mitigating stroke risk associated with AFib. To bring down the risk of stroke, you will need anticoagulants like Pradaxa, ELIQUIS, XARELTO or warfarin. These work in a way that is different from blood thinning medications used for stents. The blood thinners for AFib work by blocking small proteins called clotting factors, which help blood make a clot.

Most patients with both AFib and CAD will need both these medications since they address specific conditions related to CAD and AFib separately. However, the use of multiple blood thinning drugs can increase the risk of bleeding. However, patients with stable CAD and AFib may be able to reduce their blood thinning medications when medically appropriate per the discretion of the patient's cardiologist. This can help reduce the risk of complications when using multiple blood thinners

Patients With Both Atrial Fibrillation and Congestive Heart Failure

AFib can lead to congestive heart failure (CHF) and vice versa. With AFib, your heart rate may be too fast even when you are resting. Since the upper chambers of the heart are quivering instead of pumping blood efficiently, the heart is circulating only a fraction of the blood that it should be with each beat. The inefficient contraction of a heart in atrial fibrillation can lead to a buildup of pressure inside of the heart. This increased pressure then gets transmitted backwards from the heart to the lungs and leads to fluid accumulation in the lungs. The combination of a persistent rapid heart rate (which stresses the heart) can gradually weaken the heart, thus leading to heart failure.

I have seen many patients who develop severe congestive heart failure due to atrial fibrillation. For these patients, rapid atrial fibrillation over a period of several weeks to several months subsequently leads to a severe weakening of the overall heart function. When I first meet patients like this, I tell them that it is possible to recover a weak heart function due to atrial fibrillation, but it is a long road to recovery. I also emphasize that I will help them through every step of the way. When patients have congestive heart failure and AFib, I will frequently try a cardioversion first since it is a relatively low risk first procedure. Afterwards, an ablation procedure and lifestyle modifications will give better long-term results.

Some of my best memories of my AFib patients come from patients with congestive heart failure and AFib. There have been many patients that I have met with severely weak hearts due to AFib. Some of the best days that I have as an electrophysiologist is to be able to see that same weak heart function become normal again after treating AFib. It can be a long road with multiple steps and sometimes multiple procedures, but it can be well worth the final result.

On the other hand, congestive heart failure can also lead to AFib since it can cause thickening and scarring of heart muscle. These changes can disrupt the electrical signaling in your heart and thus lead to AFib. Patients with CHF who then develop atrial fibrillation will likely experience a worsening of CHF symptoms. Patients with both CHF and AFib are more likely to have multiple hospitalizations due to severe symptoms.

Recent literature on patients with CHF and AFib have demonstrated that aggressive treatment of AFib can significantly improve quality of life and reduce hospitalizations for CHF. There is also some evidence that aggressive treatment for AFib with an ablation procedure may improve survival in patients with CHF.

For More Information:

1. Catheter ablation in patients with congestive heart failure: https://www.nejm.org/doi/full/10.1056/NEJMoa1707855

The Athlete With Atrial Fibrillation

Previous studies have shown the complex association between endurance exercise and AFib. When endurance exercise is mild or moderate, then the risk of AFib is low. However, the relationship between endurance exercise and AFib is not that simple. There appears to be a certain limit of endurance exercise beyond which AFib risk increases.

Evidence also shows that the risk of AFib rises in a dose-dependent manner in response to endurance exercise duration. In a study on skiers in Sweden, the strongest factors for getting AFib were race times and the number of races completed. There are also other studies, including meta-analyses, that show a higher Afib risk in response to endurance exercise duration. The risk appears to be much higher for older people.

Endurance exercises can increase the risk of Afib in a number of possible ways. Although not confirmed, it is thought that the more time spent on training and structural remodeling of heart tissue as well as higher vagal tone may be responsible. In addition, there have been some studies that have demonstrated that endurance athletes who develop AFIb have increased fibrosis or scarring in the atrium. The prevalence of AFib in endurance athletes can range from 0.3 to 9 percent.

Although exercise and maintaining a healthy weight are great for the long-term treatment of AFib, unfortunately it appears clear that too much exercise is also a risk for atrial fibrillation. When I meet a patient with new AFib and a history of significant training for endurance sports, I usually counsel them that they will have to make a significant reduction in their exercise routine.

It is difficult to advise an athlete to reduce exercise, most of them are very passionate about their sport, whether that be long distance running or bicycling. Many athletes find it difficult to change their exercise routine.

It also very difficult to manage an athlete with atrial fibrillation with medical therapy. Most of these patients have a very low resting heart rate, and also most do not have high blood pressure. Many athletes cannot tolerate the most commonly used medications for AFib, beta blockers. Likewise, most athletes are very healthy and at a healthy weight, so many times lifestyle modifications do not benefit this population as much. As a result, in most athletes with AFib, procedures for AFib like a catheter ablation, tend to be the treatment of choice. Ablations can usually offer the best long-term results with minimal medications.

Young Patients Diagnosed With Atrial Fibrillation

When discussing AFib, we tend to think of it as a disease that comes with age. While it is true that the risk of AFib indeed increases with age and that many AFib patients (particularly chronic and longstanding cases) are people over 60 years old, the hard reality is that younger people are being increasingly diagnosed with AFib.

To young people, AFib comes as a shock when they are least expecting it. Although they might have conditions like stress and anxiety, they may not have any heart condition as compared to older adults or have a reason to believe that they may develop AFib symptoms. Many of these younger patients have no idea what AFib is. However, they may learn about this for the first time when they are brought into emergency care due to shortness of breath, irregular heartbeat, or any other symptom of AFib.

Obesity, endurance athlete training, and alcohol abuse are some reasons why I see AFib diagnosed in younger patients. Another common reason is sleep apnea. Sleep apnea is now extremely common among everyone, including young people, and sleep apnea is a powerful risk factor for AFib. Of course, there will also be some younger patients diagnosed with AFib where there is no clear cause for it.

Since unhealthy food, high stress, overwork, a poor work-life balance and insufficient rest and sleep have become endemic, more and more people are getting Afib at a younger age. As confounding as it might seem, Afib in young people is indeed caused and exacerbated by these same lifestyle choices. Upon in-depth questioning, younger Afib patients often concede that they have a poor diet, face excessive stress, or have little sleep (or cannot sleep enough due to sleep apnea).

Most younger patients diagnosed with atrial fibrillation cannot imagine a lifetime of this disease, and possibly a lifetime of blood-thinning medications for stroke risk reduction. For younger patients, lifestyle modifications including weight loss and cessation of alcohol use are of the utmost importance. While ablation procedures and medications may work well for the short-term, lifestyle modifications will provide the younger patient with AFib with the best long-term treatment results.

The Future of AFib Treatment

Home Monitoring Devices for Atrial Fibrillation

Since AFib is a long-term condition, you will typically need long-term treatment strategies which may include long-term monitoring. There are many long-term monitoring devices now available which include implantable cardiac monitors, and at-home devices such as KardiaMobile or the Apple Watch.

Wearing a 24-hour or 30-day external monitoring device for your doctor's office can be helpful at times but may be insufficient. People with AFib (even paroxysmal AFib) can suffer an AFib episode much later when they are no longer wearing a heart monitor. In such a case, neither they nor their doctors will be aware of what is going on. Another major problem with AFib that makes it riskier is that you can have AFib episodes without even being aware of it.

Implantable Cardiac Devices

Implantable cardiac devices are beneficial for many AFib patients, particularly those who face sporadic episodes. Such patients typically do not have another episode for a long time, which makes it very difficult, and in fact sometimes impossible, for the doctor to understand what went on during that episode. But an implantable device can capture all necessary information to give you and your doctor the full picture as to what is going on.

AFib patients who pass out due to an AFib episode will also find more benefits from implantable devices. The trouble with fainting is that it can happen very suddenly. Moreover, it is hard to tell whether the passing out was the result of an AFib episode or some other reason. Once again, with an implantable device, your doctor can accurately identify the cause of fainting and reveal if what was due to AFib or not.

Also, patients suffering from cryptogenic stroke will also find implantable devices to be of significant benefit. As you would remember from the previous discussion, a cryptogenic stroke is one whose cause is unknown. With an implantable device, your doctor will be able to determine whether or not it was due to AFib. Implantable devices can, thus, make it possible to diagnose AFib in patients with cryptogenic stroke. Without such a device, AFib might go undiagnosed if it indeed is the cause. Once AFib is correctly diagnosed, doctors can create a plan to treat it and mitigate the risk of future strokes.

Implantable devices are also of much use to AFib patients who suffer subtle symptoms. While some patients can correctly tell when they are suffering from an AFib episode, there are many who cannot. Data from these devices will help such patients to know whether they are undergoing AFib episodes or not.

When patients have an implantable device, doctors can get a warning much more quickly as to how a patient's condition is progressing. This is critical since early warning and early action is necessary for slowing down AFib progress and reducing its deleterious impact.

These devices also allow for remote monitoring to closely follow a patient's AFib. The device transmits data to the doctor's office to inform them about warning symptoms or progression of AFib. So even if patients are unaware, doctors are not since these devices keep them fully informed of patients' heart rhythms. The implantable device has an antenna that transmits this information to your smartphone, which, in turn, transmits this information to your doctor's office.

Implantable devices go under your skin, as their name implies. Thankfully, they are quite small and very easy to install. These days an implantable cardiac monitor is about the size of a paper clip. The procedure takes just five to ten minutes to get a device installed. To install the device, a cut is made on the left side of your chest above where your heart is located. The cut is small, about the size of your fingertip. The device goes into the cut and is then situated underneath your skin, above your heart. A bandage is all that is typically needed for recovery. Patients usually go home shortly after the procedure.

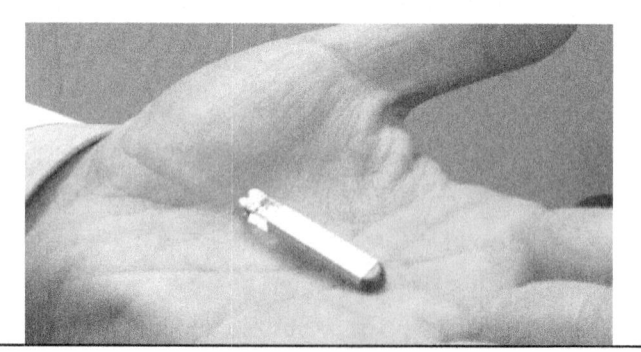

Typical size of an implantable cardiac monitor

If you have had a heart checkup before, then you may be aware of external heart monitors that doctors use to assess your heart condition. A major benefit of an implantable device is that you can go about your normal work and lifestyle without having to bother with wearing any external device to monitor your heart. This is an extremely important benefit because likely you cannot wear an external device at all times without having it interfere with your life.

The battery within an implantable device can power the unit for three years. During this time, you and your doctor will gain plenty of valuable information that can assist your doctor in formulating a viable strategy for your health and also help you to make informed choices. However, the device can always be removed prior to the three years of battery life if no longer needed.

You should get in touch with your doctor to understand if an implantable cardiac device is the most appropriate option for your needs. There are several great devices available. The good news is that these implantable devices are usually covered by health insurance. You or your doctor's office will have to check your insurance policy to find out if coverage is available.

Implantable devices, in their current form, have been around for just five years or so. They used to be much bigger than what they are now. Initial models were about the size of a finger. But thankfully, they are now much smaller, which is motivating more and more people to use them.

For More Information:

1. Learn more about the Medtronic Link implantable monitor: https://www.medtronic.com/us-en/patients/treatments-therapies/heart-monitors/our-monitors/reveal-linq-icm.html

2. Learn more about the Abbott Confirm Rx implantable monitor: https://www.cardiovascular.abbott/us/en/hcp/products/cardiac-rhythm-management/confirm-rx-insertable-cardiac-monitor.html

KardiaMobile

Wearable and at-home devices for atrial fibrillation are now extremely popular. Advanced heart monitoring devices have emerged as viable non-invasive methods for monitoring heart rhythm. Thanks to these devices, you can follow your heart rhythm in the comfort of your home, without an implant procedure.

You can purchase the KardiaMobile device for home use without the need of a prescription. When you purchase the device, you get to keep it together with all the data that it records. This, of course, does not hold true for an external heart monitoring device your doctor hands over to you, such as a 30-Day Event Monitor or a 24-Hour Holter Monitor.

These at-home devices are able to record a simplified version of the ECG that is performed in your doctor's office. Some devices are able to provide a simple, single lead ECG, while one of the newest devices, the KardiaMobile 6L, records an ECG from six different angles. As a comparison, the ECG from your doctor's office records the heart rhythm from 12 different angles. The ECG is a graph that gives a visual presentation of your heartbeat over time. Specifically, it shows the electrical activity of your heart by showing how the voltage varies with time.

By far my recommended at-home device for monitoring atrial fibrillation is the KardiaMobile and KardiaMobile 6L. The KardiaMobile devices are able to detect atrial fibrillation in about 30 seconds. You just need to put your fingers on the sensors and the device does the rest. Within a few seconds, it will indicate if your heart rhythm is normal or if you are having an AFib episode. These flexible devices also allow you to send ECG results to your doctor.

The beauty of the KardiaMobile device is that it is around three inches long, so you can keep it in your pocket or fit it in the back of your smartphone. There are two square pads on the device where you can place your fingers. It takes around 30 seconds for the device to give you the results.

With the KardiaMobile 6L, a great device got even better. The device now has the ability to record a six lead ECG, which is reflected in its name. This is a major improvement over the original single lead device, thereby bolstering its accuracy. Six leads permit a more accurate graph of your heart rhythm, which can improve the accuracy of the diagnosis. With six leads, the device can record an ECG from six different angles. Doctors agree that the six lead device is more accurate than a single lead ECG tracing.

The latest KardiaMobile device can give an accuracy of 95 percent, which is impressive for a device of its size. That being said, there are steps that you can take to further improve its accuracy and give yourself the best results.

Even the slightest movement can have an impact on the ECG since it is a very sensitive device. Hence, while taking a recording of your heart rhythm, make sure that you keep your hands stationary on a flat and stable surface like a table, for instance. This is much better than holding it in the air since even the slightest movement may impact results. You may not realize it, but hands can move in the air by a fair amount even if you are trying to keep them still. Resting the device on a surface can greatly reduce this movement for more accurate results.

In some instances, you might get an unclassified response from the device. It could be the result of poor sensing. Another possible reason is that the abnormal heart rhythm detected is not atrial fibrillation but an arrhythmia of another sort. In these situations, it is best to share your tracing with your cardiologist or electrophysiologist office to better determine any rhythm abnormality. The tracings provided by the KardiaMobile 6L are usually excellent and can be easily shared with your doctor. Any limitations in the automated algorithm can be easily overcome by having your doctor review the ECG tracings.

For More Information:

1. KardiaMobile Website: https://www.alivecor.com

2. Kardiamobile 6L page: https://www.alivecor.com/kardiamobile6l

The Apple Watch

Apple made a big splash in September 2018 when they announced that the latest generation of the Apple Watch would be able to detect atrial fibrillation through a single lead ECG.

Soon after the software update came out, there were big, splashy news articles saying "Apple Watch saves man and helps detect life-threatening arrhythmias" and other good press regarding the latest Apple Watch.

The Apple Watch Series 4 has a sensor underneath the watch which is used for not only checking your heart rate but also the heartbeat irregularity which is used for detecting atrial fibrillation. Also, when you put your finger on the crown of the watch, the watch can record a single lead ECG which can help detect atrial fibrillation over a period of a 30 second analysis.

Now, the watch itself has several potential results after the 30-second analysis. One result it could say is that you're in normal rhythm; another result could say that you're in atrial fibrillation, or you can get a notification in regard to a heart rate that is too low or too high. The last result could be inconclusive which means it doesn't fall into any of those categories that have been preset on the Apple Watch.

What I do find the most interesting about the Apple Watch is the alert system on it. It has spontaneous alerts, which is something that can alert a patient if they're potentially having episodes of atrial fibrillation, and these are alerts that you can set up on your watch for either low heart rates, high heart rates, or even irregular heart rates.

The watch itself is not constantly looking for atrial fibrillation, but if it does sense an irregular heartbeat, it can alert you and encourage you to do a proper ECG, which is, when you put your finger on the watch crown and initiate the ECG yourself.

However, the accuracy of the Apple Watch is overall unclear. I have read reports indicating a wide variety of reported accuracies. Some of the original Apple data reported an accuracy of 98 percent, however over the last two years, third-party studies have reported an accuracy as low as 34 percent. In addition, the accuracy of the device appears to be less at heart rates over 120 beats per minute, and many AFib patients experience a rapid heart rate over 120 bpm during episodes of AFib. I have also seen reports that the Apple Watch may be less accurate in people less than 55 years of age. It is possible that younger people wearing an Apple Watch may have a higher maximal heart rate which may confuse the AFib algorithms on the watch. Apple has a good reputation for making quality products, so I assume that the accuracy of the watch will improve over time.

Many people ask me, "what do you recommend, a KardiaMobile or an Apple Watch?" My answer is usually based on whatever the patient is truly looking for at that time. For someone looking strictly for an at-home monitor for atrial fibrillation, the KardiaMobile 6L is what I usually recommend, plus it is much cheaper than an Apple Watch. The KardiaMobile 6L provides excellent tracings for review with your doctor when needed. But for someone who likes smart watch technology who also wants the messaging, phone capabilities, and music options together with AFib monitoring, then the Apple Watch can be a good option.

There are multiple options for monitoring atrial fibrillation at home, however, the KardiaMobile devices and the Apple Watch are by far the most popular options at this time. Over time, I am sure new products will be released with hopefully good accuracy.

For More Information:

1. Cleveland Clinic Studies Accuracy of Apple Watch 4 for Atrial Fibrillation Detection: https://newsroom.clevelandclinic.org/2020/02/25/cleveland-clinic-studies-accuracy-of-apple-watch-4-for-atrial-fibrillation-detection/

Future Directions for Treatment Options

Much progress has been made in developing safer and more effective blood-thinning medications than warfarin that are now FDA approved. It is amazing to think that only about 10 years ago, warfarin was the only option for anticoagulation for stroke risk reduction for patients with atrial fibrillation. Overall, the newer blood-thinning medications, such as ELIQUIS, XARELTO, and Pradaxa, have shown considerable improvements over warfarin. Since the release of these newer blood thinners, they have now become the standard of care. They provide consistent blood-thinning effects and have a comparable and sometimes lower risk of bleeding when compared to warfarin.

Unfortunately, there has been little to no progress in new medications designed to control atrial fibrillation symptoms. The last anti-arrhythmic medication approved for atrial fibrillation was Dronedarone, also called Multaq, which was now approved over 10 years ago. The majority of medications used for controlling AFib symptoms, such as beta blockers, digoxin, amiodarone, flecainide, and propafenone, are all well over 20 years old.

Fortunately, there have been significant advancements made in procedures designed to treat AFib. I frequently tell patients that the equipment used in catheter ablation procedures changes every year, almost like an iPhone. There are constantly upgrades and new equipment options designed to improve the accuracy and success rate of a catheter ablation procedure.

The increasing success rate of various AFib procedures is good news for patients since these methods may reduce reliance on drugs that may have side effects in the long term. These promising new methods may have an even higher success rate then previous procedures or equipment and they may also be safer.

The catheters used during an AFib ablation procedure are constantly evolving. One of the most important features of an ablation procedure is to create thorough ablation lesions. During an ablation procedure, it is the doctor's intention to create a strategic scar to reduce and improve AFib. However, the heart is resilient, and the heart tissue may grow back despite our best attempts. Many of the equipment upgrades and new features have been made in order to provide a more thorough and consistent ablation result.

One of the best, newer features for the ablation catheters which came out a few years ago is what is called contact sensing. Up until a few years ago, there was no direct way to know how well a doctor was touching heart tissue during an ablation procedure. You can imagine it may be difficult to make good contact with the heart tissue when the heart is actively beating. These contact sensors now allow electrophysiologists to have good contact during the ablation process and has improved the efficiency of the procedure.

Another feature that is constantly evolving is the strength or type of energy used during the ablation procedure. The most traditional energy used is called radiofrequency, commonly referred to as the burning method. Heat energy is applied when using radiofrequency. There has been recent interest in using higher energy amounts at shorter durations than what had been traditionally used to improve ablation lesions.

Cryotherapy is another energy alternative which is also increasing in popularity. In cryotherapy, freezing energy is used to ablate heart tissue. AFib ablation procedures using cryotherapy have been available for well over 10 years, however the more recent generation of equipment has better success rates than the previous versions. This newer equipment has thus led to increased use of this energy type for ablation. The most commonly used equipment for cryotherapy is called a cryoballoon. In my experience, I have had good results using cyrotherapy for AFib ablations. My experience has been so good that it has become my preferred strategy for a first-time ablation in someone who has paroxysmal atrial fibrillation. I like it in this setting because I have seen good results, and it has a much quicker recovery for patients when compared to the traditional radiofrequency method.

In addition, there are also other alternative energy sources being considered, which is in an area of active research. There is some available literature on using lasers during an AFib ablation, as well as another energy type called pulse field electroportation. However, I do not get excited about new energy sources for Afib until there have been several studies confirming a benefit. Too many times I have seen excitement over a new technique or procedure for AFib, just to find out a few years later that it wasn't that good after all. Only time will tell if a newer energy sources will have better results.

Another area with frequent research is how to improve outcomes for patients with more advanced atrial fibrillation. As I have discussed several times in this book, as someone progresses with atrial fibrillation, the level of scarring or fibrosis of the heart tissue continues to worsen. It is this diffuse damage which makes it very hard to successfully reverse atrial fibrillation in more advanced cases. Over the years, there have been multiple studies looking at different ablation strategies for patients with persistent atrial fibrillation, and there has been no clear answer on a preferred strategy.

One possible reason why past studies have not yielded a positive result in more advanced atrial fibrillation is because everyone has their heart affected in different ways by atrial fibrillation. Thus, an approach which includes "every patient will gets 'x' strategy" may not be helpful for all patients with persistent atrial fibrillation.

I strongly feel that the main way to improve the success rate of an ablation procedure in more advanced cases is to customize the ablation procedure and target the most active areas of atrial fibrillation in each individual patient. Unfortunately, this is easier said than done. There have been a few methods tried over the years in an attempt to individualize ablation procedures for patients with more advanced atrial fibrillation, but none has had considerable success. There have been methods used which include what is called 1) complex fractionated atrial electrograms and 2) wavelet rotors of atrial fibrillation, and both showed promise at first. But after a few years neither option showed consistent results. Thus, the best way to individualize an AFib ablation continues to be a part of active research. It sounds like it should be easy, but these methods to individualize and target atrial fibrillation in advanced cases involves some very advanced research.

In my opinion, patients who have the best outcomes for treatment in atrial fibrillation have a three-step approach which includes symptom reduction, stroke risk reduction, and lifestyle modifications. No matter how advanced the equipment for atrial fibrillation becomes, patients will continue to have recurrences of atrial fibrillation if all three steps are not covered. No matter how great the latest feature of an ablation catheter is, AFib will likely come back down the road if lifestyle modifications and stroke risk reduction are not addressed.

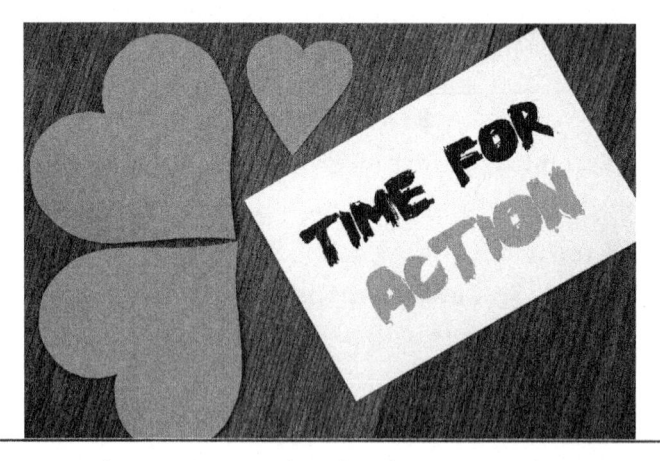

Start to take action today for better AFib symptoms.

Create Your AFib Action Plan

Now that you have completed this book, let's formulate your AFib Action Plan. Here I will help you construct a layout with which to work with your doctor to help you address symptoms for better treatment. As I recently mentioned, patients who get the best results take a three-step approach. Here I will break down these three crucial steps and help you create your own AFib Action Plan.

Step 1: Stroke Risk Reduction

As I have mentioned several times, stroke risk reduction should be the first step in treatment for anyone with atrial fibrillation. A key feature about stroke risk reduction is to understand your individual risk for stroke. Please refer back to the section on assessing your risk of stroke with the CHADSVASc risk score calculator. There are also several online calculators that will quickly give you the result of your risk score with a few simple questions. The online calculator at https://clincalc.com/Cardiology/Stroke/CHADSVASC.aspx gives a very clear result and explanation.

For the grand majority of patients with atrial fibrillation, blood-thinning medication, called anticoagulants, will be recommended. Blood thinners such as ELIQUIS, XARELTO, or warfarin, to name a few, significantly reduce a patient's risk of stroke from AFib. These blood thinners have been found to reduce risk of stroke as well as dementia in patients with atrial fibrillation. Always check with your doctor that you are taking the proper dosage of anticoagulants based on your age, weight, and kidney function. Improperly low dosage of a blood thinner, or lighter blood thinners - such as aspirin - are typically not sufficient for stroke risk reduction.

If you have had trouble with anticoagulation medication in the past, then you may be a candidate for a left atrial appendage closure procedure, such as a WATCHMAN. Excellent candidates for this procedure include patients who have had major bleeding while on blood thinners, patients who struggle with anemia of unclear origin, or patients with a significant fall risk. Check with your doctor if a WATCHMAN is the right treatment plan for you.

Step 2. Lifestyle Modifications

For many people, there are several lifestyle modifications which can make a significant improvement in AFib symptoms. In my opinion, part of the reason why many people may still experience a progression in atrial fibrillation symptoms despite medications or procedures, is because lifestyle modifications are not put in place. As I have discussed in this guide, the one lifestyle modification that has the strongest data for improving atrial fibrillation is weight loss. In clinical studies, patients that were able to lose 10 percent of their initial body weight had a major improvement in AFib symptoms.

Obesity increases risk for atrial fibrillation, inflammation, high blood pressure, diabetes, and coronary artery disease. Weight loss has shown to significantly reduce symptoms of AFib, as well as improve high blood pressure, diabetes, and overall inflammation.

Losing weight is easier said than done and sticking with it or not gaining the weight back is equally important. The best method for sustained weight loss is one where you can stick with the plan for long-term results. This is why I am not a fan of fad diets; they are usually designed for quick weight loss but may not provide long-term results. Real long-term weight loss requires time and commitment.

Likewise, it is not always only about weight loss. I have met several patients that have unhealthy eating habits and increased levels of inflammation despite a relatively normal weight. In these patients, a healthier nutrition plan can also improve AFib symptoms.

There are several diet plans that I do approve of - such as The Whole30, the paleo diet, the Mediterranean diet, or programs such as Weight Watchers. There are many excellent options out there for weight loss and improved nutrition, just avoid the quick weight loss plans or diet pills.

If you would like my help to improve your nutrition with a focus on atrial fibrillation, then check out my online program, **Take Control Over AFib**. In this online program, I will provide you with a step-by-step guide on improving your nutrition and help you implement these principles into your life with an emphasis on long-term benefits from AFib symptoms. Learn more at **https://www.takecontroloverafib.com**

With that said, there are also many other lifestyle modifications that can also make significant improvement in your AFib. Most notable would be reduction or cessation of alcohol and tobacco use.

Stress also plays a significant role in many people's AFib symptoms. As I have discussed previously, stress reduction techniques which can include yoga, meditation, or acupuncture can lead to improvement in AFib symptoms. Stress can also affect sleep quality. Putting a focus on sleep hygiene can also benefit your AFib symptoms. Lastly, I always counsel patients with atrial fibrillation to be screened for sleep apnea, as there is a strong association between AFib and sleep apnea. Proper treatment for sleep apnea can have a significant impact on AFib symptoms as well.

Step 3: Symptom Reduction With Standard Medical Therapy or Procedures

There is a reason I put this step as number three. I strongly feel that patients who put steps one and two into place first will have the best outcomes. People who only rely on medications or procedures will not likely have as good an outcome.

When it comes to symptom reduction, there are many medication options available. The most commonly used medications are beta blockers and calcium channel blockers. These are commonly used because they work well, and they are unlikely to cause long-term side effects or cause significant damage to another part of the body. However, I have also treated several patients who do not tolerate these medications; a frequent reported side effect of these medications is fatigue.

If you are experiencing side effects from these medications, please discuss your symptoms with your doctor. In some cases, your body may get used to the medication, or you may have fewer symptoms with a different medication in the same category.

One point I like to tell my AFib patients is this: you are not forever stuck on the medications you are on. There are usually many alternatives, so find the right medications that work for you.

If the commonly used beta blockers or calcium channel blockers are not controlling your atrial fibrillation, then it may be time to try stronger anti-arrhythmic medications. These medications are more specific towards treating AFib as they work on specific electric channels of the heart to slow down or prevent AFib. However, they must be closely monitored and used in the correct patient. Commonly used anti-arrhythmic medications include flecainide, propafenone, sotalol, dofetilide, and multaq.

Special note should be made of the medications amiodarone and digoxin. Both are commonly used, sometimes even used together. Although they both have a role in treating atrial fibrillation, they both have significant side effect profiles that need to be monitored closely. For both of these medications, I frequently discontinue their use as soon as possible when I feel it is safe to do so.

If you continue to struggle with medications, even anti-arrhythmic medications, then procedures may be your next best option. For most causes, I would recommend trying a traditional catheter-based ablation first. These procedures have been used for 20 years for treating atrial fibrillation and many people will have a good result. Alternative energy sources such as cryotherapy are optional depending on your circumstances.

Please keep in mind that patients who get the best outcomes from procedures such as an ablation also implement steps one and two above. A strategy for stroke risk reduction is necessary even for patients who undergo catheter ablation. Likewise, patients who get the best outcomes from an ablation also implement strategies for weight loss, reduce alcohol consumption, and treat sleep apnea if indicated.

There will be also some patients that continue to struggle with AFib despite an ablation procedure. What can these patients do next? First, in my opinion, is to make sure that lifestyle modifications are being addressed as I mentioned above, then ask your doctor if additional medications can help with residual symptoms.

If you then continue to have symptoms of AFib after an ablation, despite medication adjustment and lifestyle modifications, then you may need another procedure performed. Many people may need to have another catheter ablation procedure. In many circumstances, patients will have a better result after a second procedure. The second procedure can touch up any areas that need to be re-ablated from the first procedure, as well as identify additional areas that need to be ablated.

For patients who have failed traditional catheter ablation, or some patients with more advanced stages of AFib, they may want to consider surgical ablation procedures such as a mini maze surgery. These surgeries are typically more thorough then a catheter procedure, but also more aggressive with a much longer recovery time and higher risks. In addition, not everyone with atrial fibrillation will be a good candidate for a more aggressive surgical treatment option such as a mini maze surgery.

The last step for some patients with atrial fibrillation is the AV node ablation with a pacemaker. I frequently call this "the end of the road." I reserve this option for patients who clearly have had unsuccessful treatment despite multiple attempts at different medications or even procedures. I may also consider this option as an earlier option for some patients who I feel are too sick or too frail to undergo a traditional catheter ablation procedure. The goal of the AV node ablation is simply to control atrial fibrillation and provide a patient with a nice, steady heartbeat with the help of a pacemaker. But as I mentioned previously, after an AV node ablation is performed, a patient is dependent on a pacemaker for all their heartbeats for the rest of their life, which is why I usually reserve this treatment option as a last resort.

Conclusion

As you complete this guide, I hope that I have provided you with the necessary tools to feel like an empowered patient. I hope that now you have confidence when it comes to your atrial fibrillation. Reduced symptoms, reduced risk of stroke, and multiple treatment options are all available to improve your individual symptoms.

Remember, atrial fibrillation is a chronic condition, so make sure to keep this guide handy for future use. Features of this book which may not be pertinent to you at this time may become more pertinent to you in the future regarding your care.

Atrial fibrillation is long-term condition, so make sure that your treatment strategy focuses on long-term success. Short-term strategies without a long-term plan will inevitably result in a recurrence of AFib. I hope this book has helped you imagine the tools that you will need for long-term success.

As the years go by, newer treatment options will likely become available. Newer treatment options may include medications or new procedure equipment or techniques. Hopefully, one day, advances in atrial fibrillation will result in a true cure for atrial fibrillation.

To stay updated on the latest treatment options for atrial fibrillation, follow along with me by visiting my blog at **https://drafib.com.**

Sign up for my email list or connect with my social media pages. Here you will stay updated on the latest treatment options and connect with a community of like-minded patients striving for better care and improved symptoms from atrial fibrillation.

As you continue your path living with atrial fibrillation, I wish you nothing but the best when it comes to your treatment. I hope that I have helped you develop the tools you will need to get the best treatment possible. Let us all strive to improve atrial fibrillation together, one day at a time.

Printed in Great Britain
by Amazon